PRAISE FOR

THE BOOK WE WISH WE HAD

———

"This book is an incredible story about the most important job we are bestowed in our lifetime; having relentless perseverance to protect, love, and raise our children to realize their fullest potential. I really do wish I had this book when my kids where young."

—John R. DiJulius III Author of *The Relationship Economy*

"Lisa's book has the PERFECT title. If you are a parent navigating a terrifying and medically frustrating experience, wouldn't it be invaluable to have a resource steeped in moving stories and sage advice that helps you feel less alone? Not only does she bring the reader into their personal experiences through raw detail, I dare you not to get goosebumps from her storytelling."

—Kelly Lafferman, CMO & Principal Findsome & Winmore
and Registered Mental Health Counselor Intern

"This book is a powerful testimony and roadmap for parents in need of navigation for neurodivergent children. Lisa's brave and unfiltered story shows us how mental health is a journey for families, school systems and communities alike so we can create more loving and inclusive environments that allow all children to thrive."

—Shannon Green, former *Orlando Sentinel* columnist and Editorial
Board member, mom to a child with Tourette's, ADHD and anxiety

"Lisa Bachman's story brings powerful support to others facing terrifying and bewildering challenges as parents. She guides readers through a dark, frightening tunnel to the light at the end. I've seen Justin speak on stage, demystifying this taboo subject with humor and honesty. This book is told from an extraordinary mother's point of view. It offers honesty, hope and healing and will help many parents through their own journeys."

—Lucy Boudet, Parent

"If you are looking for a story that represents all the good in the world, then *The Book We Wish We Had* is perfect for you. It is a reminder that with the right people in our corner, anything is possible."

—Brad Cohen, Assistant Principal, Author of *Front of the Class: How Tourette Syndrome Made Me the Teacher I Never Had*

THE BOOK WE WISH WE HAD

THE BOOK WE WISH WE HAD

How We Stayed Hopeful
When Hope Wasn't Enough

LISA BACHMAN

WITH JUSTIN BACHMAN

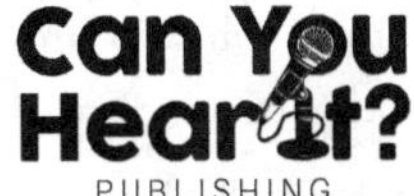

This book is dedicated to…

The officials from the Boardman Cross Country race on September 18, 2010, and the Ohio High School Athletic Association. It if weren't for your denial of Justin's diagnosis, we wouldn't have come as far as we have!

Acknowledgements

The writing of this book has been a journey and a dream come true. It has been more than a two year effort that would never have happened without my supporting cast. I do not have enough words to thank my husband and soulmate. Ron, you walk behind me to catch me when I fall, in front of me when I need protecting, and by my side every single day. Your belief in me is endless and your love for me is truly unconditional, and I'm thankful for it every day of my life.

Stefanye and Konnor, growing up for you was tough, and you made many compromises because so much energy was focused on the darkness of mental illness that sucked the life out of many rooms. Yet you never complained. To say you are my heroes is an understatement. Stef, you were our compass, guiding us when the experts couldn't. You jumped in with wisdom well beyond your years to organize our lives in a special way. Konnor, your approach taught me more than you will ever know. You brought the calm after every storm. Your ability to step back and see the big picture always reminds me that the bad times will pass. Matt, we are so thankful to have welcomed you into our family, and are another calming factor bringing logic and love. Wyatt and Max, you have given us the gift of the special world of being a grandparent. Its far better than anything we could have expected.

Ron, Stefanye, Matt, Konnor, Justin, Wyatt and Max—I love you past the sun, moon, and every star in the sky. You bring sunshine into my life every single day.

Joanie Schirm, your insistence that our story be put to paper is the reason this book happened. You knew the idea was in my head and you gave me the confidence to put it to paper. You didn't simply tell me to write. You coached me, made connections, and encouraged me daily to make this dream a reality.

Alice Peck. Thank you isn't enough. You took my words and worked your magic to help me weave a compelling story. We would not be where we are today with your guidance and tender care. This book is better because of you.

Lucy Boudet. My soul sister. You read a very early version and your honesty gave me the confidence to write something that could actually help people. You showed me how to believe this could be something helpful and you helped me find my voice. I am eternally grateful for your friendship.

Linda Mullen and Nancy Brady. You are both amazing friends who talk me down from the ledge on a regular basis. You are my confidants, and the support you provide is an incredible gift.

Shannon Green, you have been my go-to parent. Watching you raise your children has motivated and inspired me. I've run concepts from this book by you, and your feedback has propelled me forward.

Libby Moore. I'm not sure where to begin, but your helping me learn to love and appreciate me for who I am as a person propelled me forward.

Mandy O'Dell. You brought our dream to visual life by designing this amazing cover! Your brilliant design skills nailed it in the first round. Your generosity has touched our hearts, and we will be forever grateful.

Duane Stapp, thank you for walking us through the publishing process and ensuring every I was dotted and every T crossed.

Crystal Sershen, thank you for your eye for detail in ensuring the editing of this book made sense. You went above and beyond to help us further develop the story.

To you, the reader of our story. Thank you. Thank you for purchasing this book and journeying alongside us. We are not the experts, but we hope you can glean something from our journey that is helpful to you as you navigate your own maze.

Justin—this was a labor of love, and there are no words to describe the pure joy it was to work on this project with you. I'll miss the calls where we worked together to review the stories and go back and forth to ensure we picked just the right words. We did this and I'm so proud of us!

Table of Contents

Justin's Letter to His Childhood Self

Dear Justin,

You are in the middle of your darkest days. Let this letter be the light at the end of your tunnel. You will get through this. I remember the spot you're in way too well—thinking I had nothing to offer and being so convinced the world was better without me. You tried to die three times but thank God you weren't successful. You have way too much to contribute to the lives of other people to ever consider ending your own again.

You're dealing with a lot right now. Your body is fighting against you, and you don't understand why. You'll figure that out pretty soon—it's this crazy disorder called Tourette Syndrome. That's why you always make that little "hm" sound that drives you crazy at night. It's part of the reason you can't sit still at your desk. Right now, it's why you hate yourself.

I know you tried to jump out of a second-story window.

I know you tried to jump from the top of the bleachers in the school gym, hoping the crudely painted basketball court on that smelly rubber floor would be the last thing you ever saw.

I know you believe you mean nothing, but I promise you that's not true.

You're about to meet a woman our family calls Mary Poppins. She's going to save your life. Seriously. I don't quite know how she did it, but you're going to start to be okay with your quirks and differences. She will help you control your anger, help you learn how to make friends, help you stop hating yourself for being yourself.

This may sound impossible. I remember how we used to think. Nobody understood. Nobody cared. That feeling of worthlessness defined us for a long time, but it's completely false. You are going to save lives and make changes bigger than you can possibly imagine.

I just got back from a meeting at a high school. It was about a boy named Nico. He's a few years older than you are now, but he's dealing with some of the same stuff. The meeting was the same kind that Mom and Dad went to with principals, coaches, band directors, and teachers to figure out what to do about you. Nico is struggling like you are. His differences make learning and school incredibly difficult. Much like Mom and Dad, Nico's parents are amazing, supportive, and willing to move heaven and earth to help him, but they don't know what he's going through. That's where we step in and help. Right now, you may think you're worthless, but if you ask Nico's parents, we are changing the world.

We caused a lot of trouble, especially in elementary school, and Mom and Dad didn't really know how to handle it at first. You're going to go to special classes, there are going to be people called "interventionists" whose job is specifically to watch out and make sure you are safe and doing okay. Things will start to get a little better. Those thoughts of wanting to die will diminish, and eventually you will get diagnosed with Tourette Syndrome. Although a scary-sounding condition, it will come as a relief because then you'll be able to get answers.

Somehow, in their hearts, everyone knew we weren't a bad person: you and me. You're just lost, looking for anything to grab hold of to feel normal. I'm sorry to be the one to tell you this, but normal is something we never really achieve. As scary as that may sound, it's actually a good thing. Once you get diagnosed with Tourette's, you'll feel great. You will finally be able to explain those weird sounds and movements, and eventually you'll become a motivational speaker because other people will want to hear your story. (This still blows my mind.)

I know that a few weeks ago you looked Mom in the face and told her you wouldn't live to turn eighteen years old. You told her you were a worthless kid, and you would die before that changed.

You could not be more wrong.

I know how deeply you believe that, but I have some wonderful news to share. I am writing you this letter on May 10, 2019. At twenty-one years old, I will graduate from college tomorrow with a degree in journalism. We chose journalism because of a strong belief that everyone has a story to tell, and that those stories matter.

More than anything, you are worth it. It's going to take you a long time to realize this, but once you do, nothing will stand in your way.

Tomorrow, I don't walk across that stage to graduate and get my diploma.

We do.

As much as I hate how much I used to hate myself, you and I are equally important to this journey.

We have saved lives. We have changed worlds.

I know you won't believe me. I never wanted to believe anyone because I thought nobody understood. I see a lot of that in Nico, but I know he'll come around, just like you will. It's going to take the hardest work you will ever have to do, but once you get through, it will all have been worth it.

I am so proud of you. You've got a long way to go to get to that stage tomorrow, but you are going to make it! Once you do, you'll look back at your life and ask how in the world any of it was possible.

To be completely honest, I still don't know how we made it out alive.

All I know is that I'm glad we did.

I love you,

Justin

We Dared to Dream

There was a time when we never dared to dream. At all.

For most of his childhood, our youngest son had no friends. Justin was never invited to birthday parties or bar mitzvahs. A playdate at a neighbor's house was a rare occurrence. Justin was *that* kid, the one nobody wanted to be around. Teachers dreaded having him in their classes. Moms and dads called the Little League administrators to make sure their children were not put on a team with Justin. We were those awful parents who could not control our child.

It was a dark time. People judged us. Well-meaning friends recommended we "Get Justin a few sessions with a psychologist and he'll be fine." They accused us of being helicopter parents and said we needed to give him space.

How do you not *hover over a child on suicide watch?*

You can never leave a child on suicide watch alone. Ever.

Hope is nice, but it isn't enough. I lost hope more times than I can remember. It was faith, powerful love, relentless work, and sheer will that got us through four life-and-death crises with our son. One the result of illness at birth, the other three by his own hand—attempted suicide. Before the tender age of 11 years old.

I thank God every day that we found Justin before he could follow through.

He was our child. Even though he didn't believe in his worth, my husband Ron and I did, and so did his sister and brother—Stefanye and Konnor. We had no choice but to help him. The problem was that we had no idea how. There was no map to follow. Parenting books didn't cover this. And (especially at first) there was very little support.

Nothing.

The one thing I knew was that we would do this together, as a family.

For years, Justin's challenges engulfed us. Ron, Stefanye, Konnor, and I each shared the responsibility in our own ways. Our life was a maze. We'd travel down a path, hit a wall, and be forced to turn around and find another way through. Soon, blazing paths became our specialty. We were determined to never give up on Justin or our family. Along the way, we lost a lot of people we believed were our friends and supporters. We felt alone, forgotten, angry, and terrified. There were tears, fights, dread—you name it. Every ounce of our patience, marriage, and confidence was tested. *Everything.* But we had each other. The five of us. We even came up with a slogan: BGOD—Bachman Gang or Die.

Depression, anxiety, autism, Asperger's, Wilson's disease, oppositional defiance disorder, bipolar disorder, executive function disorder, paranoid schizophrenia, severe allergies—these were all the misdiagnoses Justin received before he was eleven years old. It wasn't until he was twelve that he was given the proper one—Tourette Syndrome with coprolalia and dystonic tics accompanied by ADHD and OCD. Once we knew the correct path to follow, our lives started to get better. That's why we call Justin's diagnosis of Tourette's our gift—it explained so much and allowed us to learn, adapt, and most important, advocate.

Now, ten years later, my heart is beating with anticipation.

I'm crying. But the tears are no longer ones of fear and sorrow. These are joyful, full of love and pride. I'm sitting with my family in the Carrier Dome getting ready to watch this incredible human, Justin, walk across the stage at Syracuse University's Newhouse School of Public Communications, where he will graduate with an amazing job as a broadcast journalist. He is going to report the news—Tourette's and all.

As we entered the Carrier Dome, professors shook our son's hand and students called out to Justin to say hello. *He has friends.* People wanted to sit with him, were asking him to hang out afterward. *He has a future.* To them, this was natural, but they had no idea of the true depth of this accomplishment.

Ron, Konnor and I take photos to send to Stefanye and Matthew, as they were too far along in their pregnancy to make the trip. We're beaming with pride, watching Justin cross this stage and reflecting on the hundreds of stages he has crossed with a passion for sharing his journey not only to live, but to save the lives of others lost in the darkness he once inhabited.

Joining us in spirit are a host of characters who helped along the way. I laugh out loud remembering the day our very own Mary Poppins opened her umbrella and floated into our home in Cleveland, Ohio. I smirk thinking about the cross-country officials who disqualified Justin because they deemed him "rude"—if they only knew how their cruelty backfired and sparked a blaze of success. Most of all, I think about the twenty-nine young people who didn't die by suicide because they believed Justin's message.

This is *our* triumph. It feels like all five of us—the whole Bachman Gang—are graduating.

Moreover, it is Mother's Day. There could be no better gift.

This book is our story. It is dedicated to all the kids and adults who feel alone because no one understands what they're facing. It is for all the parents worried about their children, the siblings who are lost, the teachers who don't know how to handle a student, the healthcare professionals who are uncertain how to respond to a patient. It is for friends who are fearful or unsure what to do, and for anyone who simply feels "other."

This is the book we wish we had.

THE BOOK
WE WISH
WE HAD

CHAPTER 1

At the Brink of Life and Death

"We are going to do everything we can."

"What do you mean?" I asked the Chief Resident at Rainbow Babies & Children's Hospital.

Everything you can to what? Everything you can to get him out of the ER today? Everything you can to get the right doctor? Everything you can to give us answers?

She looked at me like I was nuts—like I should have known precisely what was happening. There was a younger resident in the room who stepped up and kindly said, "Your son is gravely ill. We are not sure what this is, but we need to do some tests. Right away, because his life is in danger."

Whoa.

Wait. Did I hear that correctly?

A freight train headed right at me.

Justin's life was *in danger.*

My baby was only seven days old.

Now what?

Shit.

I looked over at my husband. Ron was as stunned as I was. Neither of us could speak. I couldn't even cry. I didn't know what to do; my thoughts raced. In the five minutes we waited for the doctor—an eternity—my mind went places no mother should ever have to go.

I'd always wanted four children.

Both Ron and I were excited about number three. We had moved into a bigger house, and we were ready. The pregnancy was great. No issues, routine testing, no morning sickness, the usual tiredness—not a big deal. We opted to let the gender of the baby be a surprise, and were excited for the big reveal at birth. We got our older kids involved. Stefanye was seven and Konnor was four. We had fun betting on whether the newest member of the Bachman Gang would be a boy or a girl.

I was one of three siblings and always felt like the odd man out, and I didn't want that for our kids. Stefanye and Konnor were close, two peas in a pod. When I got pregnant with number three, I was sure there would be a number four.

But now, our baby was in jeopardy.

On June 8, about six weeks before I was due, Ron and I, our kids, and a couple other families went out for dinner. About an hour after we ate, I began to feel off, and soon became violently ill. I had food poisoning. I was so sick and so far along in my pregnancy that my water broke. I noticed that the amniotic fluid had some green in it and recalled hearing from either my doctor or Lamaze instructor that this meant the baby had pooped.

By the time Ron got me to the hospital, my nausea had settled. Even though I wasn't having contractions, the doctor wanted to give me some time to let things happen naturally. This seemed odd, but she assured us I was far enough along that everything should be fine. This was the same obstetrician who delivered Konnor and Stefanye, and she was the only one I'd ever had, so I had complete faith in her—both Ron and I adored Dr. Greenfield. I was tired, and I was nervous about the baby coming early, but I also felt that thrill—Number Three was on the way, *and* I was skipping the last long month of my pregnancy!

By morning, I was still not having contractions, so the OB team induced me and about an hour later, we welcomed our beautiful son Justin Parker into the world. He appeared to be perfect!

Three days later, Ron and I brought our baby home, and we felt like old pros. We had done this twice before. We knew the ropes. We didn't have the nerves we had with our first or second. Plus, we had helpers! Stefanye was totally prepared to be the second mom and was so happy to be supportive. She could not wait to sit and feed little Justin, hold him, and do all the things a mommy does. He didn't really cry that much, so she felt expert at this job.

I didn't see it then, but I know now—*what baby doesn't cry?*

Konnor was fascinated with Justin. He would sit and stare at him, but Konnor was much more interested in Power Rangers at this age. In fact, he was absolutely certain he was going to grow up to be the Blue Power Ranger. Konnor told Justin story after story about his favorite superheroes.

During the first days after we brought Justin home, there was a lot of activity in our household. Because he was early, the nursery was not finished. Because he was a boy, we had to plan a bris—the traditional Jewish circumcision ritual that takes place at eight days old. Friends and family gather to celebrate and welcome the child into the Jewish family. During this ceremony, the baby is also given a Hebrew name. We were planning to hold this celebration in our house, and we had only five days to finish the nursery, pick Justin's Hebrew name, and prepare and cook for this grand event for over fifty guests.

My mother is an artist, and she got busy painting a Dr. Seuss scene on the nursery walls. Stefanye wanted to be her helper, so my grandmother came to care for the baby while Ron and I did all the things we needed to do. I remember thinking Ron and I really had the hang of this parenting thing because Justin was so easy, but we were so busy and excited that we didn't notice he was sleeping too much.

How did I miss this?

The day before the bris, my grandmother sat in the rocking chair, holding Justin. It occurred to me I had not fed him in a while, but he was sleeping so contentedly that I figured he would wake up when he was hungry. Another hour went by, and he was still asleep. At this point, I was in pain and needed to nurse, so I figured, "Okay, kid—you need to eat!"

I took him from my grandmother and joked with her because he was so warm. I told her she was the best cuddler ever because the baby was so cozy! When I sat down to feed him, I could not wake him up. I grew concerned—not panicked, just thought *Hmm, he really is tired.* But he hadn't been up much in the night. I said, "Okay, little guy, you need to eat," and I rubbed his head. It was *hot.* That's when it dawned on me that this was not body heat from snuggling Great Grandma—it was a fever. I found our thermometer and took Justin's temperature. It was 106! This was extremely high, especially for an infant.

I called our pediatrician because I wasn't sure what dosage of Tylenol to give. I definitely did not expect him to tell me to get this baby to the hospital right away. So much for my pride in being a "chill" mom. The doctor called the hospital and told them to be ready for us.

Although I knew this was serious, it never occurred to me it was dire. Stefanye and Konnor had recently had strep, so I figured Justin must have caught it. Worrisome, yes; needed action, yes; but I believed the doctors would check him out, prescribe an antibiotic, and send us home in a few hours. This was more of an annoyance and an inconvenience. After all, if he were that sick, wouldn't he be crying and miserable? I told myself he was going to be fine.

Ron had gone out for a jog, and I wasn't sure when he would return. I tend to be good in crisis situations—as long as there is no barfing, I can handle it. While I waited for him to get back, I made a to-do list with the last-minute stuff I needed for the bris. My mom was still at the house, so she could take care of the kids.

Although it felt like hours, Ron finally arrived. I tackled him the second he walked in the door. Didn't even say hello—just, "The baby is sick, and we have to get to the hospital." It felt like the trip to the

ER was something to check off my list so we could get back home to finish our plans—after all, we had about fifty people coming to the house the next day.

Ron and I tend to be yin and yang. I was busy with my to-do list, so he took on a concerned role and wondered if this was more serious than we realized. One of his home repair customers happened to be the Head of Pediatrics at Rainbow Babies and Children's Hospital, so Ron called him from the car and asked for advice. Dr. Avner told him we were doing the right thing, to follow our doctor's instructions, and that he would check in on us. We didn't know it then, but Dr. Avner was a kidney specialist, and we were going to really need him.

When we got to the hospital, we were greeted by the Chief Resident. She didn't have a great bedside manner and was bossy, but I ignored that part. My only concern was, "Take care of my kid." A younger resident told us the Chief Resident would do an initial exam and that we were welcome to sit in the waiting room. *Um, no.* There was no way we were going to leave our sick seven-day-old baby's side. So, I let the Chief know we would be staying. We got a bit more attitude from her, but this was just noise, and we ignored it. She did all the typical things doctors do, then she looked at us and matter-of-factly said, "We are going to do everything we can."

Think about being the mother of an infant and hearing those words: *We are going to do everything we can.*

Ron and I froze, waiting for her to finish the sentence. *Everything you can to what?* To select the right medicine? To make sure he isn't miserable? The grim expression on her face made my panic surge. I finally gathered my words, "Everything you can to *what?*"

To this day, more than twenty years later, I can close my eyes and be in that exact moment. I looked over at Ron, and he was stunned, eyes full of tears, unable to speak. Yin to his yang, I shifted into Mama Bear mode.

The younger resident told us they had a strong suspicion this was bacterial meningitis, and the best way to diagnose it was to draw spinal fluid. They needed our permission for a spinal tap, and I gave it, but we were not leaving our baby's side. The Chief Resident began to do the test, and she was having trouble. The younger resident tried to correct her, but the Chief Resident would have none of it.

I could feel my anxiety rising. I told her to stop. Our baby was screaming in distress, and it was clear to me the younger doctor knew what to do, but his superior was insulted. She became angry, yelled inappropriately at the younger resident, and let me know that I should not be questioning her credentials. The Chief Resident was a cold bitch as she informed me that the younger resident was not qualified and that she was going to do this. She triggered my defense system.

Remember that Mama Bear mode? My "bitch switch" flipped.

I looked at her and spoke in a quiet but firm tone, "Not only will you not touch my child, but you need to leave this room." I turned to the younger resident and asked, "Do you know what to do—do you *really* know what to do?"

"Yes."

A power struggle ensued. The Chief Resident was intent on having things her way, more interested in being right than helping a sick baby. At this point, our pediatrician—Dr. Worthington—walked in. I looked at him and said, "Get her out of here." I was livid; I was scared. He could tell I meant business and he asked her to step out. She complied, the junior resident did a fine job, and the spinal tap was on its way to the lab.

That's when I asked, "What is bacterial meningitis?" The doctor began to explain, but the only thing I recall him saying is that a child this young and small had only about a 2% chance of survival. I heard nothing after that. It didn't matter.

Dr. Worthington told us Justin would need to be admitted to the hospital and he would be back in touch in the morning to confirm the test results. Because they strongly suspected meningitis, and because of its aggressive nature, they would begin treating it proactively. Ron and I settled into the hospital room, and the gravity of our situation struck us.

By now, it was late at night, and we were hungry. We looked at each other—we were lost. We had one question and one question only: *Is our baby going to die?*

CHAPTER 2

Our Rights as Parents

The nurses were fantastic. They saw our zombie-like state and could tell we needed some direction. They asked us when we had last eaten. We could not remember. Neither of us wanted to leave Justin's side. One of the nurses suggested we call and order a pizza that could be delivered to the room. Thank goodness for delivery! Baby steps.

We called home to check on the kids and let my parents know we were staying at the hospital. We reached out to two friends and asked them to help us cancel the bris. This kind of information travels fast, so we didn't need to do much.

Ron and I held each other and cried. We were petrified we could lose our beautiful boy. There was nothing to say, so we sat in silence. Neither one of us got any sleep.

The next morning, Ron's customer Dr. Avner came into our room. Ron is good at relationships, and he had fostered a beautiful one with both Dr. Avner and his wife, Jane. Dr. Avner was a nephrologist, which meant he was a kidney specialist. He told us the test results were positive for bacterial meningitis and that there were E.coli bacteria in Justin's kidneys. He repeated the words, "we are going to do everything we can." There was that phrase again.

How can this be happening?

But Dr. Avner was encouraging. We were grateful for his calm demeanor and appreciated his reassurances. Yes, the situation was grave, but he told us that we were in the right place, making all the right decisions, and doing all the right things.

He encouraged us to see the positive signs. After a few hours of antibiotics, Justin started crying more—this was the best sign! Although not eating well, he was eating. His limbs were moving, and we were told to celebrate every wet diaper because this meant the kidneys were working!

So, of course, poor kid, I was constantly checking that diaper—never in a million years did I think pee would bring me so much joy.

My mind was overloaded and overwhelmed. I felt helpless and out of control. I searched for a reason this was happening. Was it the poop in the amniotic fluid? Yes—that must be it! Then, something else popped into my head—food poisoning. I had food poisoning and passed it on to my son.

Ron and the doctors thought I was blaming myself, but I wasn't. I was looking for an explanation. I didn't eat bad food on purpose.

To cope with this, I had to hang onto something logical, something that made sense.

Being the "all business," serious type of person I am, I asked about the treatment plan. We knew Justin was sick, but we were not going to accept that he was going to die. We were going to fight. This was our child, and because we were warriors, it was in his genes to fight. Dying was not an option. We were hanging on to that 2%, and we were determined to focus on anything favorable.

By our second day in the hospital, Justin was moved from neonatal intensive care to the stepdown division for small babies. Although born early, Justin weighed seven pounds, six ounces at birth and his lungs had fully developed—one of those good signs! But the illness and treatment would bring his weight down into the four-pound range, and his critical condition required twenty-four/seven monitoring.

Bacterial meningitis is a disease that attacks the major organ systems in the body. This meant we had many doctors on his care team. We had

Infectious Diseases, Nephrology, Urology, Gastroenterology, and a few more "ologies" thrown in.

Of course, every doc had their own opinion on the right strategy. One would come in and order some test or treatment, and then another would come in, disagree, and write orders to change the plan. I felt like someone put a blindfold on me, spun me around twenty times, and expected me to figure out how to hit the bullseye.

Nurses brought medication. Sometimes it was because the IV bag was empty, but other times, it was because a doctor ordered a change. I quickly realized I had to question everything. I could not just accept when a medication was changed; I had to know why. I had to know what was wrong with the old one and what the new one was going to do. I had to ask about side effects. Our baby was so tiny, and these drugs were so strong. The names of these meds were so long and foreign—not ones I could easily remember (or wanted to remember!). I wrote everything down.

Part of me felt bad about challenging the nurses. I gained a huge appreciation for them because they are caught in the middle. They had confident doctors telling them what to do and uneducated parents making demands. Our nurses were saints.

Then there was the diaper rash. This may be TMI, but our poor baby's butt was fire engine red and bumpy. He would scream at the lightest touch. There was no such thing as a normal bowel movement. That wouldn't happen for almost a year. We called it Dijon mustard. (*Eww*…right?)

Early during the hospitalization, I asked one of the nurses if the medications were impacting Justin's eyes. They always seemed to be rolling to the back of his head. My internal alarm went off again when she rushed out of the room. It turned out these were seizures. I felt like someone turned my world upside down again. We added a neurologist to the team of specialists.

I was barely getting any sleep through all of this, and the fact that my son was now having seizures added another level of fear. Would he be brain damaged? Babies at a few weeks old don't do much but sleep. This was normal, but I had no normal. I didn't expect him to smile at this age, but I wanted his eyes to track my movements. *Nope.* Not happening. I wanted him to squeeze my finger. *Nothing.*

The nurses told me to sleep when Justin slept, but that was too scary. I had to be reassured that the monitors attached to his body would pick up changes in his breathing and immediately notify people who were watching for alerts.

Stress. So much stress.

There was a pamphlet titled "Patient's Rights" in our room. At first, I didn't pay attention to it. I figured it was some sort of advertisement. But one day, I just so happened to pick it up—a sure sign of my boredom—but wait! This was a good pamphlet! It told us to exercise our patient rights. And we did. We demanded a meeting that included every single doctor caring for Justin. We needed these people to get on the same page because we didn't care what mountains they had to move, they were going to move them, and they were going to do it together. The squeaky wheel gets the grease, and I was squawking!

On the fourth day of Justin's hospital stay, the summit was held in a large conference room. A doctor from each discipline was in attendance. They started talking in medical jargon, which may as well have been a foreign language.

There was a white napkin in the middle of the table. I watched my husband stand up with the intention of commanding the room. In a bold and sweeping gesture, he threw that napkin in the air the way a football ref throws a penalty flag. Then he yelled, "A penalty has been called on the field." Everyone stopped talking and looked at Ron. He has a sarcastic, sense of humor. He has a way of making everyone laugh just when you need it most. This was his moment. He got on his "pedestal" and requested that the doctors please speak in English so we could understand what everyone was saying. Somehow, we were going to have to make sense of all the things each of these expert doctors were saying so we could figure out a care plan for our son. If we were going to bear the responsibility of consent for treatment, we had to know and thoroughly understand our options, because our son was not going to die.

Thankfully, Ron's stunt lightened up the room, and progress was made. This meeting lasted three hours. By the end, we were so thankful for these medical professionals. Three hours is like eons to them. Medications were selected, and timelines were drawn with measurements to see if they were working. We had a plan!

At least for a while.

The medicines Justin received were strong, and he was tiny. The diaper rash was bad, but it was nothing compared to what the drugs were doing to his little veins, which were slowly breaking down. This meant the nurses had to continually move the location of the IV. It was in one arm, on his hand, on one leg, then the other. Those were not bad, but when they had to insert the needle into his neck, then his head—well, that made me hurt along with him. When all was said and done, the IV locations would be moved to twenty-seven different parts of his body. I felt every needle stick in the exact same place they stuck him.

But I had to be strong. During each procedure, I put my face close to his, so our skin was touching. I would sing to him to make him feel better. Thankfully, having two older kids, I had a good repertoire of classics, like "Hush Little Baby" and a plethora of songs by Rafi! And, if I could not remember the words, I made them up.

As each IV location was changed, Justin cried more and more. Dr. Avner's words echoed in my head—this was a good sign! He was fighting. I became his cheerleader, encouraging him to yell. *Yell your head off and keep fighting!* When he would cry, I would yell along with him.

Eventually, after the twenty-seven IV punctures, the doctors decided to do a surgical procedure to install a catheter. This was a version of an IV that was put into his neck and went straight to his heart.

A baby's heart is about the size of an olive. Let that sink in for a moment.

The surgical procedure and was done under sedation in an operating room. Giving anesthesia to a baby that young, and that sick, is high risk, so after the insertion, a nurse stood in the room with me, essentially watching Justin breath. After four hours he was deemed safe, and it was determined that the monitors would suffice.

That was not enough for me, so for many more hours, I stood over the isolette and continued to watch him. I was not able to hold my baby because they needed to keep him still, but I was vigilant. I stood and watched his chest rise and fall. For hours. Eventually, I told myself he was fine. The nurses were coming in frequently, so I gave in and opted for a little sleep. I had just drifted off, when all of a sudden, alarms were blaring, lights were flashing! Before I could even sit up, there were ten people in our room with a crash cart.

I froze.

I couldn't move.

What is happening?

Why are all these people here?

I can't see my baby.

The alarm kept blaring—surely the entire hospital heard it.

I'm out of my body.

No one was answering me.

My baby's heart stopped.

Is he breathing?

I'm going to puke.

Then, after less than thirty seconds, they left. Apparently, one of the monitors disconnected and signaled the desk that Justin's breathing had stopped. A false alarm.

I burst into tears and cracked up laughing all at once. I didn't know what to think.

There was no need to be scared because in reality, nothing happened.

I went into the bathroom, threw up, and went back to bed.

After about a month, we started to feel comfortable with Justin's improvement. We didn't know how this wicked disease would impact him, but that didn't matter. We felt that no matter what life was going to hand us, we would be able to deal with it.

He was going to live.

CHAPTER 3

Living in the Hospital

I moved into the hospital with Justin. Ron and I decided that this was the best solution. The doctors told us that my nursing him would give him the best possible chance, so I stayed. Through our time there, there were rays of sunshine and funny moments.

I didn't have a lot of visitors because Justin was just too sick, and although it was summer, we didn't want to risk anything. Ron brought me a nice dinner every night, and when we finally felt it was safe, he brought the kids to see their baby brother. We had picnics on the floor and made it as much fun for Stefanye and Konnor as we could. I played games with them and did the best I could to be their mom too.

Ron was very honest with Stefanye and Konnor. We didn't want to frighten them, but we told them their little brother was sick and the doctors were taking care of him. We let them ask questions, but they really didn't have any. With Stefanye at age 7 and Konnor at age 4, there was no way they could truly comprehend the enormity of what was happening. (I know we couldn't get our head around this, so how could they?) We assured them Justin and I would come home, and they believed us.

At these ages, scheduling was important for Stefanye and Konnor, and Ron did all he could to keep their life as normal as humanly possible. He got them up and out the door to go to camp every day and made sure they had time with friends. They would have family dinner together, and in true Ron fashion, laughter was always on the menu. Ron played with

Konnor and his Power Rangers, and he helped Stefanye with her hair. He polished her nails and even let her polish his nails!

Looking back, I have no idea how we handled this or how we knew what to do. Ron was coming to the hospital as much as he could, but he had to bear the burden of taking care of our kids, and, because he owned his own company, he only earned money when he worked. I always said it was harder on him because he was driving back and forth to a hospital thirty-five minutes from home. He typically came in the morning after dropping off the kids and hoped to get there for doctor rounds. Sometimes he made it, but occasionally he didn't, and I would do my best to translate.

He also had to deal with answering questions from family and friends. Often, we didn't feel like talking, but we knew their curiosity was out of care and concern. Everybody wanted to know what was happening. We always did our best to put on our brave faces to keep those close to us updated. But it was a burden. Everyone thought we were so strong—everyone but us.

I learned that the things I appreciated most were the people who just did something. My family was there for us. My parents helped Ron by preparing meals, doing our laundry, and keeping the house picked up. My mom stayed with Justin while we had our "doctor summit," because we didn't want him to be alone.

People sent muffins to the hospital for me to share with the nurses. This was awesome, because the hospital staff was so helpful. It allowed us to do something when there was only so much I could do myself. Our babysitter, who happened to be a counselor at the kid's camp, knew the kids needed to be picked up from camp at the end of the day, so she called and simply told us she would take care of it. Sadly, I had been so distracted that I had not considered who would pick up the kids—thank goodness our sitter did!

Some of the people who felt helpless sent cards or would call and leave a message, letting us know they were thinking of us. I especially loved it when they left the message and indicated there was no need to return the call—what a relief! There were some people who were frustrated when I didn't return their call. I felt bad, and certainly didn't mean to ignore them, but I didn't have the energy and wished they could understand. Every ounce of brain power was on my son's care.

Even though so many people rallied around us, I still felt isolated. We were hospitalized over the July fourth holiday. I sat by the window in my room, thinking about all the people who were having fun—enjoying picnics and watching fireworks. My husband and kids were at a friend's house. I know Ron did not want to go, that he wanted to be with me, but we were trying to make things as normal as possible for Stefanye and Konnor. I had a realization that so much is done for people in the hospital on Thanksgiving and Christmas, but not on the other holidays. I made a promise to myself that I would do something to change this.

Living in the hospital as I did, I made friends with the staff. Because we could not have visitors, I needed to lean on these people. I was so lucky that I had a steady flow of workers in and out of our room. I knew the day nurses, the night nurses, and the weekend crew. I made friends with Mary, the woman who brought my breakfast and lunch trays. I would hang out with Nancy, the woman who cleaned our room. She would come in every morning with the brightest smile and say, "*Giiiiiirl…* How are you doing today?" She was consistent—every day, same thing.

Justin was hospitalized in June, which is when the new crop of residents rotates in. The one assigned to us was named Angela. Dr. Angela. She played such an important role, not only in Justin's care but in mine. Angela was new to Cleveland, and although she knew the other residents, she didn't know anyone else. We bonded. At the end of her shifts, she would come in and talk with me—like a friend. I got to know her personally, and she got to know me. I only wish I could tell her how much of an impact she had on our lives, as our busy schedules did not enable us to stay in touch.

The tests Justin needed to ensure his treatment was working included collecting his urine. It could not come from a diaper because it had to be totally clean. The only way to gather it was to take off his diaper and be ready to catch it. The first time we had to do this, Angela came in and explained the process. I laughed because I could not figure out how this would work. Looking back, I should have held him up so she could put the cup under him, but why do something that makes sense? She was new, and I was oblivious! Justin lay on his back, we took the diaper off, and both of us stared at him. Angela held a cup. At first, nothing happened. We stood there, and I suddenly got the giggles, imagining how silly we looked. Since the giggles are totally contagious, Angela started laughing too. We were laughing so hard, we were crying! Of course, that's when Justin started to pee, and we were so busy cracking up, instead of catching the pee, we got a beautiful golden shower. It was comic relief sorely needed.

Another special person I met was Toni. She was the social worker assigned to me. Yes, me. Thankfully, the team at the hospital knew that although I was not a patient, I needed care. Toni was so kind and helpful and talked me down from the ledge on more occasions than I can count. She helped not only with my psychological wellbeing, but acted as a translator of sorts. We would meet daily to review Justin's progress, and Toni helped me formulate questions to ask the doctors. She also navigated Ron and me through the mountains of paperwork from hospital bills and insurance.

Eventually, we began discussing the plan to go home. I was petrified. As much as I wanted to be in my house and in my bed, there was a huge sense of security in having the doctors and nurses right there. Although Justin's heart never stopped, what if it did? Would we know what to do? There were so many things happening, and he needed so much care, would I be able to handle it when I was alone?

I was about to find out. After eight weeks of being in the hospital, it was time to go. When you go to an ER or have an outpatient procedure done, they give you "going home" papers. After having been there for months, we got a book. There was a lot. Not only did we have medications, but we had to be vigilant about developmental milestones. There was a concern that Justin's hearing might be impaired as a side effect from the medications, and it was possible he would have other problems, ranging from kidney issues to discolored teeth. His food schedule would be different because his tummy was a mess. But we were prepared. We had a plan! I never wanted to be caught off guard again.

We learned a lot from this hospital stay, and I know the universe lined it up to prepare us for things to come. Ron and I learned we were lucky. We were a team that worked together. I was strong during the hospital stay and held him when he cried; he was strong when we got home, and I fell apart. We gained confidence as parents because we were able to take care of our older children and we made sure they knew they were loved and an important part of what makes our family work.

We learned that doctors are not gods and that we had to ask questions. *We had to.* No one knew or cared about our child more than we did, as parents, and we had to ensure every single angle was considered, every scenario thought through. And, when someone didn't cooperate, like that Chief Resident, we learned it was okay to ask for someone else.

We learned the importance of advocating for ourselves. There is a subtle difference between fighting and advocating but one that makes a big difference in a successful outcome. It's a tightrope!

The most important thing we learned was that there were bad days, really bad days, but there were good ones too. If we didn't laugh, we would always be crying. It was up to us to find the silver linings. They are easy to overlook, but they are there.

What we didn't know, as we packed Justin into his car seat to take him home to be with his sister and brother, was that our lessons were just beginning.

CHAPTER 4

A Home and Classroom Disrupted

The doctors told us to expect many physical impairments, but aside from some developmental delays, they didn't materialize. Justin had no urinary tract infections, no stomach ulcers, no hearing loss. It was Justin's mental health that would prove to be our enemy.

None of us slept much during the first two years of Justin's life. His body needed to normalize and recover. It took about a year before his digestive system worked properly. Some days, he screamed so loudly that our neighbors who lived three doors down would come over to make sure he was okay.

Our biggest worry at first was that Justin wasn't walking. Stefanye and Konnor were both running by a year old, but not Justin. All his motor skills were lacking, but the doctors reassured us he would catch up. Justin took his first steps a few weeks before his second birthday.

The one thing that was *not* delayed was Justin's speech. The kid talked nonstop, and he was *loud!* In fact, he was so loud that we suspected something was wrong with his hearing, but no…he was just loud. (He still is!)

This was a precursor of things to come.

Dr. Avner's advice stuck with us, and we looked for every positive sign we could find. One of my favorite memories of Justin's first two years was our bedtime ritual. After we'd read a book, I'd turn out the lights and let him talk until he tired himself out. Then came my favorite part—the goodnight kisses. First, a kiss on the cheek. Next, we rubbed our noses together, and then butterfly kisses where our eyelashes fluttered together. No matter how good or bad the day, this was a ritual that continued for many years and created something for me to hold on to.

Once Justin started walking, his toddler years were pretty typical. We were so happy he was healthy that we didn't notice some of the signs we should have addressed. He had boundless energy and curiosity. He would ask a million questions about everything, all day long. It was exhausting, but we were so thrilled his brain was working, we never tried to turn the dial down on the energy. Discipline didn't happen.

The autumn after Justin turned three, we enrolled him in the Montessori school where my Mom taught. We put Justin in her class because it was a familiar, safe environment. He had some play dates, and even met a girl he was certain he was going to marry. They asked for a stove as their wedding gift.

He became the typical pain-in-the-ass little brother to Stefanye and Konnor. Justin drew all the attention from the room. Stefanye tried to discipline him, and Konnor ignored him.

In our minds, we were enjoying typical days.

Yes, there were tantrums, sibling rivalry, and arguments, but nothing seemed out of the ordinary. Life was good.

Our respite wasn't long—first grade at public school was a different story.

Justin was unusually smart. That curiosity of his earlier years meant he had a wealth of knowledge his peers had not gotten to yet. He would try to turn a game of kickball into a science project when other kids simply wanted to kick the ball. He'd obsess over the angles and the way to bend his feet as he kicked. The result? He was always the last one picked...if he got to play at all.

We didn't notice the cues when this was happening. During those first weeks of school, he would angrily say things like, "No one wants to play with me." And I'd dismiss this by saying, "Of course people like you! You are a great kid." I'd launch into all the things that made him special.

Looking back, I realize I didn't listen to him. I wish I had asked a few more questions to understand what was really going on. If only I'd asked, "What makes you think no one likes you?"

Sadly, his first-grade teacher was no help. The calls started in October. Behavior we saw as energetic, she labeled disruptive. Where we described him as "curious," she called him a "know-it-all." The teacher confirmed the fact that the kids were not including Justin, and now we were forced to believe him. What kind of message did we send to our son—we believe you now that the teacher confirmed it?

During that first phone call, she took it upon herself to diagnosis him with ADHD and demanded we get him on medication. This caught us by surprise, so we asked for a meeting with the teacher and the principal. We didn't know either of them well. Neither Stef nor Konnor had been in this teacher's class, and neither of them had any reason to interact with the principal.

To say that meeting didn't go well would be an understatement. When I tried to explain Justin's sense of curiosity to Mr. Principal, he looked at me and said, "Mrs. Bachman, every parent believes their child is brilliant, but yours is simply a behavior problem."

How dare he call my child a behavior problem!

Mama Bear roared. I was not going to tolerate what I deemed insensitivity. I was going to protect my cub at all costs. I still saw Justin as a sick child who needed protecting, and I was not ready to admit he might have behavioral challenges. It was a mistake I can see now, but I couldn't see then. At the time, Mama Bear explained to them that Justin was smart and it was their job to mitigate the playground problems and find a way to stimulate him academically.

Ron was a bit further along than I was in accepting we might have a problem, but he let me advocate and I appreciated that we stayed on the same team. After the first meeting and the many that followed, he would kindly offer suggestions on how I could have handled the situation in a more positive way. Sometimes I welcomed them, but mostly, they irritated the hell out of me. That was how we rolled.

Although I know I could have acted in a better way, I wish the teacher and principal had known how to manage me as a parent. I they wish had been patient and talked to me in a way that helped me see what the classroom looked like when Justin did the things they described. If only they had used specific examples and talked with empathy to demonstrate they understood how hard this was for Ron and me to hear. Indicating they recognized my point of view might have calmed Mama Bear and allowed me to listen better. They could have given us our dignity and let us know they had our child's best interest at heart. All I could see was a teacher refusing to listen. She dug in her heels. She was emphatic that Justin's energy was not energy, but ADHD. By the end of the meeting, we agreed to have Justin evaluated and left it at that. A compromise was reached.

We were so humiliated that we were "called to the principal's office" that we never asked what services were available to us. It wasn't until Justin was in fourth grade that we learned our rights as parents and that this was a service the school was supposed to offer us. They had a psychologist on staff who could have done the evaluation. Instead, they sent us off to have this done by our own private doctor at what was for us a huge expense—$1,300.

We took Justin down to the Cleveland Clinic, where their team did the extensive evaluation and told us exactly what the teacher suspected—a diagnosis of ADHD. I had a really tough time reconciling the teacher's awful treatment with the fact she had been correct. In retrospect, I realize I should have gone back and had a conversation with her. After all, she was right, but her message was lost in her method. I was still so angry about the way we were treated that having a meaningful conversation simply did not cross my mind.

Ah yes…the gift of hindsight.

We took all our paperwork from the school and Cleveland Clinic to our pediatrician so we could figure out our next steps. How were we supposed to handle this new phase of parenting? After much discussion, we opted not to put Justin on medication, but to work with a psychologist.

We were worried about putting our child on meds. We'd heard rumors about Ritalin and Adderall, and we were not comfortable making this our first choice. With all his past medical problems, we were worried about adding medication that might hurt his kidneys. We wanted to give the psychologist a try.

This did not go over well with Justin's teacher, who would regularly call me, insisting—even begging—that we put him on meds.

This pissed me off.

What right did this teacher have to tell me what to do?

I got that he could be a "disruption"—but isn't she supposed to know how to deal with him?

How dare she try to tell us how to raise our child.

We were not willing to turn Justin into a lab experiment.

And let's face it, who was this all about? The teacher or our son?

Couldn't this teacher just show a little kindness? We had just received an upsetting diagnosis, and not once did she ask how I felt about it—no, she kept harping on how it would make her life easier if he were medicated.

Couldn't she respect that we were trying? We were doing the best we could and wanted to attempt counseling first. Couldn't she give us even a tiny bit of credit as parents for doing what we thought was right for our child?

It seemed cooperation was not an option.

If only she had presented us with ideas on how to work together to help him.

Her viewpoint and words were hurtful. She had her mind made up—our son was bad, and we were making him worse. Sadly, she took our disagreement with the teacher out on Justin—he was constantly penalized.

I was so angry. I didn't know what to do with this anger, and that made things bad. My anger turned to hate, and that was worse. It's hard to come back when you have hatred in your heart. It stops you from seeing the big picture. I now had tunnel vision, so this teacher didn't have a shot at doing anything right because no matter what, I was not going to see it.

More important, this sent Justin's self-confidence into a downward spiral.

He was not making friends. He had several friends in preschool, but no more. Gone was the safe environment with a caring teacher.

We were starting to have some challenges at home too. Although homework in first grade was minimal, it was always an argument. His motivation to do things was low, resulting in more arguments. I would ask him to help set the table for dinner, but he had no interest. If I nagged him or tried to discipline him, it turned into a tantrum. It became easier to not ask him to do anything. I didn't realize how much I was enabling him. He got out of helping because I didn't want the war to begin.

But we still had our bedtime routine. Those kisses meant everything.

We started working with the psychologist. We went to the office together, and she would call Justin in and either Ron or I would stay in the waiting room. Ron and I did have some "check-in" sessions with her, but they were all pretty much the same. She felt Justin was making progress—that was all we heard for the first two years.

Looking back, we should have realized sooner that the work with the psychologist wasn't doing much. But Justin seemed to enjoy going. We mistook his willingness as a positive sign. I wish I had realized that no change, and in fact, worsening behavior meant the therapy was not enough. Just because the psychologist was nice didn't mean she was the right fit for us.

We hoped second grade would be better. Justin was assigned to Mrs. Drip, a teacher we knew was awesome. I had volunteered when Konnor was in her class, so we already had a strong relationship. We were certain life would turn around for Justin.

Unfortunately, this was not the case.

Mrs. Drip quickly developed a dislike for Justin. He was a nuisance in her classroom, and she had no patience for his energy.

Justin's handwriting was poor. We attributed this to his early illness and that his motor skills had not yet caught up to where they should be. But Mrs. Drip wasn't having it and essentially decided that Justin didn't care. He would turn in his work, and it would come back with the word "sloppy" written in red letters and circled for emphasis. His grades continued to decline along with his attitude.

We were baffled at how such a great teacher could be so callous. It never occurred to her to dig into this more, that he wasn't a bad kid. At eight years old, Justin had a reputation with the teachers, and he couldn't shake it.

How do you live with that?

I was beside myself with frustration.

Justin expressed his anger in many different ways. He was great at the "death stare." He would often add to this glaring stink eye by making a fist that he would put on either side of his head by his eyes. His pointer fingers would pop out to ensure you knew he was looking right at you. If he was really mad, the other four fingers would pop out and also point at you. If he was really, really mad, he would put up one foot and point his toes in your direction. This seems funny, but if we made the mistake of laughing, it fueled his fire.

One day, Justin opted to direct this finger-pointing dance at Mrs. Drip. This did not end well. She marched him to the principal's office and told the staff he needed to be sent home. Which they did. Unfortunately, this turned into her "go-to" strategy. Pretty much every day, I would get a call and be told to come pick him up. It was a huge disruption to my day. My company was growing, but I had no choice. He came first.

This coin had two sides. The first was payday for Justin! He hated being in school and was smart enough to know that if he misbehaved, he could get himself sent home. On the flipside, he knew he was "bad," which caused him to sink deeper into depression.

Now, add the other children in the classroom to the mix. The kids knew that if they triggered Justin, something would happen to interrupt their school day. What kid doesn't want a break? Occasionally, they even got an extra recess so Mrs. Drip could "deal with" Justin.

Was this bullying? I've really struggled with the use of this term. The definition of bullying is: unwanted, aggressive, repeated behavior that involves a real or perceived imbalance of power. This was happening. Other kids had a perception of power, and triggering behavior was constantly being repeated. This definition applied to the teacher too. How upsetting is that?

Mrs. Drip became annoying. She would call us with petty things, like the day she called to tell me Justin was "excessively using tissues," and she wanted me to send in more boxes.

Seriously, excessive tissue use?

Did she really say that to me?

Yup.

This was so odd because Justin wasn't sick, and I didn't see any "excessive tissue use" at home.

I asked him about it, and he told me Mrs. Drip made him blow his nose whenever he sniffled, which he deemed to be very annoying.

Bullying? Maybe. Did I really have to deal with this? I had so much on my plate—Justin, two other children, a fulltime job.

Mrs. Drip made the complaint, so we had to address it.

Neither Ron nor I noticed the sniffling, until we paid attention. He was in fact sniffling, but he was not sick. We called our pediatrician, and he suggested we take Justin to an allergist. Off we went to what would be the first in a series of appointments that sent us down the road of incorrect diagnoses.

The allergist said Justin was allergic to fur, but we didn't have pets.

The doctor saw a tendency for seasonal allergies, so we put Justin on allergy medication.

Nothing worked. The sniffing continued and we learned to not pay attention to it. Maybe this was Justin's subconscious way to get attention? All I knew was I was not going to let sniffling become an issue. We figured if we ignored it, it would go away. If Justin was doing this on purpose, we were not going to reward him for this behavior. If you don't acknowledge it, he will stop. Right?

If I could go back in time, I'd kick myself—not too hard on this one, but we didn't pay enough attention. It was the first sign of many about what was really happening with our son that we would completely miss.

Besides, we had other things to worry about.

Justin was constantly acting out and calling himself stupid. He would say things like, "nothing matters" and "you hate me—everyone hates me." This was not typical behavior for a second grader. His anger was growing. We talked with the psychologist, and she labeled his anger as "storms." She tried to help him recognize his anger and then to take deep breaths.

We didn't see it, but Justin was slipping into a dangerous depression. The work with the psychologist wasn't enough. She tried to tell us we needed to put Justin on medication, but we were not ready to listen. We should have.

Ron and I were also starting to butt heads. Although we never blamed each other, he always said I was too lenient, and I insisted he was too tough. These disagreements would continue for the next several years, but for a long time, we didn't address them. We would argue and move on. After all, arguing had become a family dynamic.

My company, All Points Connect, had just earned a great contract with the Cleveland Indians to help with their fan entertainment. I hired a group of high school and college students to provide face painting, T-shirt tosses, hot dog tosses (can't make that up!), and other fun activities. There was one student who stood out. He introduced Ron and me to his parents, and as luck would have it, they ran a youth football league called the Solon Saturns. It was our town's tackle league, and we knew this would be perfect for Justin's energy level. They typically started kids in third grade, but agreed to start Justin in second grade.

He loved it. He was the smallest kid out there and somehow ended up at the bottom of every pile, but as the layers peeled off, he always bounced up. Ron coached his team, and this turned out to be a wonderful release for Justin. It was only for a few months each autumn, but it was a respite.

Justin would take his stance on the defensive line and growl at the opponent—his growl was so loud, we could hear it in the stands. The growl became a joke among parents, but in a good way. By the biggest stroke of luck, he didn't get hurt for four years. He would go on to continue playing through sixth grade, when his football career ended with him being carried off the field with a broken leg.

I want to say he made friends, but he really didn't. The other players liked him as a member of the team because he was pretty good and he was tough. But they never called him to play outside of football. This was hard. All he wanted was one friend, but that one friend was nowhere to be found.

Not even one.

Even though we all found respite at the games, and we so badly wanted football to make a difference for him, it had little impact on our overall situation.

We had some tough decisions to make.

We decided to investigate medication before Justin started third grade. We agonized over putting him on Ritalin. The psychologist was in favor of it, but our pediatrician was not. He was concerned about the side effects. Justin was on the lower end of the growth charts, and a big side effect was a reduction in appetite.

We did research and sought out other people whose children had taken it, but we quickly learned this topic was taboo. Justin being on medication would be our secret.

Although he wasn't for it, our wonderful pediatrician agreed with our decision to give Ritalin a try. Our compromise was to start with the lowest dose, beginning two weeks before school started so we could watch him. I was petrified. I worried he would stop eating, stop growing, and have other side effects of this drug. But we plunged in. My solace came in the fact that we were trying the lowest dose possible.

The first day he took it, we saw immediate results. His demeanor was much calmer and he seemed more able to focus. I felt better and told myself this was temporary—just until he got over the hump. Our hope was that the medication would give him the ability to get something out of the sessions with the psychologist and when he learned how to use the tools, he would go off the meds.

At this point, Stefanye was about to begin tenth grade, and boy was she organized! She was such a godsend to me—more helpful than she will ever realize. She helped Justin pick out his school supplies and worked with him on a color-coding system for each subject. She assisted him as he organized his room with labels, so everything had a place. She was so fantastic; it was a gift. Little did we know this was the beautiful beginning of her career as a special education teacher.

We had a plan—third grade would be great!

Justin's new teacher, Mrs. Matthews, exceeded our expectations in every way. She was kind and took an interest in Justin. She came to watch him play football! We were so excited—a teacher who was willing to work with us and cared about our son! She made us feel like good parents—so different from his other teachers. Instead of calling me out and making me feel bad, she worked with us.

Just wow.

Mrs. Matthews went the extra mile to see that Justin's poor hand-writing was not behavior, but something more. She realized that Justin was smart, but was perplexed over why he was failing his tests. Math facts were a big deal in third grade. They did timed tests of the multiplication tables. Justin rarely finished and always failed. Part of this was because his numerals were illegible.

Instead of calling him lazy, she opted to try an experiment. She gave Justin a verbal test. She put on the timer and asked him the math facts. Not only did he get 100% of the answers correct, but he finished before the clock ran out. I still remember her calling me to tell me the great news.

I cried tears of joy. Never before had a teacher called me with good news about Justin!

Mrs. Matthews consulted with the school's occupational therapist, and they suggested we get Justin evaluated for dysgraphia.

In dyslexia, people see things differently. In dysgraphia, people write differently. It is a disorder causing dysfunction in the coordinated effort of the brain to communicate with the motor skills needed to write and use proper grammar. For example, Justin always wrote the letter S sideways. Words would be spelled backward, and his handwriting was messy. So messy, in fact, that it was not readable.

Ron and I were somewhat relieved about this because we knew we could do something about it if this was the case. There was an answer—typing.

Back to the Cleveland Clinic we went.

The doctor at the Clinic recommended we put Justin on an IEP. We had no idea what that meant and learned it was an "Individual Education Plan" and a mandate for students with disabilities.

Hearing the word disability was hard.

Disability.

Disability.

It made no sense. He was smart, how could he have a disability?

In fact, his intelligence would prove to be a barrier. School officials would assume that because he was smart, he didn't need help. But he did have a disability.

Disability.

I would repeat that word in my head, simply not wanting to believe it but having to believe it.

Shit was getting real.

We had to face facts.

How could we use this word with Justin? He was smart enough to know it wasn't "normal," so how could we tell an already fragile kid that he wasn't normal?

So, how did we do it?

Well…we didn't.

We never used the word disability. We told him we were going to get him help with his handwriting. We were getting pretty good at this denial thing.

Based on the doctor's recommendation, we requested an IEP from the school, but we were told that Justin did not need one because he was so smart. Instead, they put him on a 504 plan that would provide some limited services with the school's occupational therapist.

We could live with this. He wasn't on the "disability" plan.

Given his behavioral problems, looking back, we should have pushed for more. But we didn't. We still saw this as a phase. To deal with things, I often whispered to myself, "This too shall pass."

I still believe in that phrase, and I use it today; however, back then, I was not letting myself see the enormity of our problems. It's really hard to admit when you have a problem, and even harder when your child does.

The school gave Justin a device called an Alpha Smart, which was essentially a keyboard with a printer. He could type his responses to questions, and we hoped this would result in better grades.

Having to use the Alpha Smart got Justin curious, and one day while we were driving to the grocery store, he asked, "Mom, do I have a disability?"

I froze.

Do I tell the truth or do I lie?

Think fast!

Will I crush his spirit if I am honest? But how can I lie?

I told him that yes, he did have a disability, but that we were working hard to figure it out. I told him the Alpha Smart was one of those tools to help him.

He went silent. I had no idea what to do. I tried to talk to him, but he wouldn't answer. I got fearful that this would launch a storm, but thankfully, it didn't. We drove the rest of the way, saying nothing, and he followed me through the store like a zombie.

I was devastated. I felt like I had broken my son—again.

Years later, Justin would tell me he hated the Alpha Smart, that it made him feel alienated because he was the only kid who needed a keyboard. I wish I had asked him how he felt about it. Maybe, just maybe, we could have explained things better. I decided it was helping, so it didn't matter how he felt. I wish we had given him some choices so he could have come to the decision to use the tool on his own.

But the Alpha Smart *did* help. His teachers were able to read his work. We had our struggles with it, but it was a tiny ray of sunshine despite the negatives.

Although academics were getting better, Justin still had no friends at school, and things at home were bad. The number and intensity of arguments was growing. Those damn fingers would pop out daily. The humor in the stink eye was long gone. The "storms" rolled in at a moment's notice. Justin was constantly lashing out at all of us for the smallest of things.

Some nights I would go for my routine of goodnight kisses, and he would turn away from me and not speak. His darkness and silence spoke volumes. Those kisses were the thing I held onto and now, I couldn't even get them. I treasured the nights he was willing to connect and cried on the ones when he would not.

He never knew I cried.

No one did.

Not even Ron. Well, maybe he knew, but we never talked about it.

On the outside, we acted like a happy family. Embarrassment would never allow us to show how much we were going through. I considered myself a strong person and therefore, no one needed to know what was happening behind the closed doors of our house.

Nobody knew I wasn't happy.

Nobody knew I was so worried about all my children that I had constant headaches.

Nobody knew I loved my husband with all my heart, but we were always fighting.

Nobody knew I was falling apart, little by little.

The biggest problem was that I knew it, but I pushed myself to the back burner.

I held things in until I couldn't. The person who got the brunt of it was Ron. Every argument sounded similar—me exploding and Ron asking why I didn't say something sooner.

I was so tough with all the teachers, but I couldn't tell anyone how I was feeling. I could, however, tell everyone what they were doing wrong and how they should be fixed, but I needed fixing too. I stood up and fought for everyone but myself.

When Halloween rolled around, I volunteered to help with Justin's classroom party. He loved dressing up and went as Darth Vader. When I got to the school, all the kids were milling about the classroom, laughing and having fun, but Justin was sitting with his head down on his desk. Mrs. Matthews said he seemed a bit blue that day and she was letting him be by himself. I went over and sat down next to him, and he told me no one wanted him to join in because he was stupid.

My heart broke.

I wanted to go ask every kid why they were excluding my son.

I held back tears and tried my best to encourage him to go be with the other kids, but the only thing he wanted to do was march in the parade. That was going to have to be enough. The risk of a storm was too great.

Later that night, Ron took Justin trick-or-treating, only Justin and Ron. Stefanye and Konnor had gone out with friends, but we tried not to impose and have their little brother tag along with them. A storm was brewing.

CHAPTER 5

Lightning Strike

The next day, lightning struck more violently than ever before.

Through all these storms, Justin would get violent, but it was never toward other people. He never tried to hurt anyone other than himself.

Except for once—on that day, he went after me. This would be the one and only occasion he would ever do this. He pulled out a steak knife and told me to back off or he would hurt me.

I was stunned.

What do I do now?

My nine-year-old son is pulling a knife on me.

Shit. Fuck. Shit.

(I don't typically swear, but when I do, it is because I mean business.)

I was petrified.

Frozen.

I didn't know what to do.

Thankfully, Ron, Stefanye, and Konnor weren't at home.

I used words and calmly tried to talk him down. I tried to placate him. I told him he didn't want to hurt me.

"Yes!" he screamed. "I do!"

The more I talked, the more wound up he became. He was in a rage, and it seemed almost as if he had left his body. The knife dropped out of his hands, and he thrashed on the floor as he shouted and yelled.

This is what his storms typically looked like. He yelled really loudly, and his ears turned the brightest shade of red. He stomped his feet as he marched around and flailed his arms, knocking down anything in his path. Sometimes he would bend his knees, as if to get his entire body into the intensity of his yelling. Then he would often drop to the floor and roll around in a fury of rage and then get back up and yell some more until he was worn out.

No one knew what this looked like. Only our family saw these storms. If we saw one coming when we were out in public, we were quick to remove Justin from the situation to the privacy of our car or anyplace else. Stefanye and Konnor often retreated to their rooms when the storms rolled in, and who could blame them?

During the Halloween Storm, I had the idea to send him out of the house to the garage. It wasn't public, so the neighbors wouldn't know, but I knew, and I knew *he* knew that he had been kicked out of the house. I even locked the door so he couldn't get back in. I yelled through the door that he would stay out there until he calmed down.

This wasn't as misguided as it might sound. One thing I had learned about his storms was that making Justin cry would bring the release of emotions that could bring the storm to an end.

So I continued to yell terrible things about how he would regret his behavior, and I screamed that he had to stop yelling. I didn't realize I was modeling the exact behavior that needed to end. I made it about me. But I knew he had to get through it too. I wanted calm for him just as much as I wanted it for me.

Well, he showed me! Justin picked up a baseball bat and began pounding on the door. Because it led from the house to the garage, it was a heavier, metal door, so he put a lot of dings in it, but it was too strong to be broken.

I let it happen.

I was desperate. I would do just about anything to get relief.

For some strange reason, the garage seemed like a safe space. He was out of the house and isolated. Never did it occur to me that this was the most dangerous place of all. There were tools in there—lots of tools. Thank goodness he never realized these could do more damage than that baseball bat.

Eventually, on his time, Justin started to cry.

I also hoped that kicking him out would make him realize the enormity of his actions.

Nope.

I thought I was doing the right thing—that getting him out of the house and into the garage would help.

I guess I wasn't thinking either.

These fits of rage were severe, and Justin wasn't conscious of what was happening to him. The anger took over with such an intensity that he couldn't process anything. He was literally out of his mind. The best way I can describe it is like a seizure.

But once he cried (and he cried *hard*), his emotions shifted to a horrible sense of guilt.

On the afternoon of the knife incident, he finally came to me, and I hugged him tight and listened to him verbally beat himself up. He called himself every name in the book—stupid, dumb, worthless. And he was exhausted.

Even though I was angry, I was more relieved the storm was over, which is what allowed me to be able to hug him. No matter what, I loved him.

We ended every storm with butterfly kisses. It was our thing.

My hope.

My salvation.

When Ron arrived home from work, the storm had passed. Justin was upstairs in his room. I told Ron the story and that we needed to have a talk with Justin—he could never pull a knife on me or anyone ever again.

Together we walked upstairs, opened the door to Justin's room, and saw something we will never forget.

____

CHAPTER 6

Good People

The room was a mess. Justin's clothes and toys were strewn all over the floor, as if he had opened every drawer and tossed everything out. This was typical. He always threw things when he was angry.

The difference this time was that the window was wide open, and he had pulled off the screen. He was perched in the window well, dressed in his taekwondo uniform with a pillow under his shirt. He was about to jump!

Our little boy looked directly at us and said, "I'm leaving the world. I don't want to live in it."

I could not comprehend what I was seeing. I held my breath and felt every nerve ending fire.

My mind raced in a million directions.

Did he really mean this?

Was the pillow meant to save him?

Did he not realize he could have broken bones?

Is that why the pillow?

Was the "it" death?

Was he looking for attention?

Did he believe his life would end?

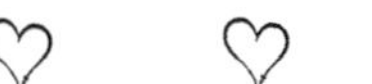

This was Justin's first suicide attempt.

Ron and I knew what it was, but we didn't want to admit it. We didn't want to say the word. We shared an unspoken communication that this was serious, but we shifted into denial. Justin was only ten years old. This was too young for him to have been serious about anything. He had no idea what he was doing.

We were wrong.

We did what we thought was best. We sat down on the floor among the ruins of his bedroom, and we talked. We told him things. Things like:

"Hurting yourself won't solve the problem."

"Hurting Mom won't solve the problem."

"You always have regret after you have these storms, so don't do it again."

"Why do you do this when you know you will feel bad after?"

Although we believed we were saying the right things, we were not. A year from then, with the help of therapy, we would finally learn how to talk with our child.

But not that day.

Suicide.

We knew what it was, but the word was taboo, so we didn't say it.

We didn't admit it.

We couldn't believe it.

We didn't want to believe it.

We had no idea our denial was setting us up for something worse.

Justin knew what he had done was wrong, and he felt awful. He told us he was too much trouble for us and that we should not have to deal with him. I will never forget what he said next: "You are good people, and you should not have to deal with me."

He called Ron and me "good people." What child calls his parents "good people?"

Deep in our hearts, we recognized the signs. We didn't act on them. We should have taken his words seriously and we should have immediately gone to a hospital. But we didn't.

We went on doing things the way we had been doing them. There was more yelling. A lot more yelling. And there were tears. So many tears. The storms continued to intensify. The garage door sustained a lot of damage and so did our family dynamic.

They say the definition of insanity is repeating the same action while expecting a different outcome. We did the same things over and over, but they did indeed change.

They got worse.

———

CHAPTER 7

Too Close

It got to the point where there were no good days. The Bachman Gang walked through life like robots.

One Sunday in late March, I heard stomping and screaming. *A storm.* Ron and I looked at each other, hoping that the other would say, "I'll go." Clearly neither of us wanted to deal with this. But based on the noise we heard, both of us decided to head upstairs.

Justin and Konnor had their own bedrooms but shared a bathroom. Each side had a set of light switches and apparently, Konnor had been in the bathroom and flipped the switches, so they were not all pointing in the same direction. This caused Justin to launch into a tirade. He started yelling that we didn't care what he wanted.

I'm stupid.

What I want doesn't matter.

Nobody cares.

You are better off without me.

Pretty much the same things he said every time.

Of course, we again immediately told him that wasn't true, and we attempted to reassure him. The more we assured him, the more enraged he became.

Broken record.

Not this again.

Helpless.

Hopeless.

Fear.

Give me strength.

God, please give me strength.

What we didn't realize was that his self-esteem was so low that Justin believed we were lying. It would take us another year before we figured this out.

After about an hour of shouting and reasoning, we put him in his bedroom and held the door shut. He would pull it open from the inside, and we would pull it closed from the outside. I was afraid one of us would cut off a finger. When he eventually realized we were not letting go of the door, he backed away, and we heard him throwing things around and stomping. Eventually, after what seemed like forever, the room got quiet.

Ron and I sat outside his door, heads in hands, crying. We were both shaking, we felt so helpless.

We were waiting for the right moment to enter Justin's room. We figured we would go in when he started crying.

We waited.

Suddenly, we realized the room was too silent. This was new—he was never quiet.

We listened really hard because surely, he must be walking around, throwing something—because if he wasn't doing that, he would be crying.

We waited. Noise would start any minute.

The quiet continued. Simultaneously, we looked at each other with extreme panic and barged into the room.

We opened the door to Justin's second suicide attempt.

This was even uglier.

This was shocking.

Total disbelief.

We dropped to our knees with a helplessness we had never before known.

Justin had clearly put more thought into this since the last attempt. Apparently, our telling him he would not have died during the last try was the only thing he'd learned. The silence was him hatching a better plan.

There was no pillow.

No protection.

I believe the human brain is a great self-protector. Ron and I blocked out details that we did not want to remember, but we cannot deny they were there.

What I saw when we walked into the room was a wide-open window with no screen. Justin was sitting on the floor, and he had pulled the sheets off his bed.

He was quiet, he was focused, he was busy. His ten-year-old brain was engineering his hanging. One end of the sheets was secured to the bed. It looked like he was planning to propel himself out the window with the other end secured around his neck.

That was my assumption. I could not bring myself to ask him what he was doing.

There was no need to ask, because I knew.

I didn't want to know. Neither did Ron.

But we did.

We caught him in the nick of time. He wasn't physically hurt yet.

Yet.

Too close.

If we had waited another minute, maybe two, this would have had a different outcome.

The difference sixty whole seconds can make.

There was no ignoring anything this time. We had to use the word; we had to do something.

What do you do when your child doesn't want to live and you can't process the enormity of it all?

We had to face facts. This was a smart kid. He knew exactly what he was doing.

He was so young that the mechanics didn't matter. He had an end-game. He was able to visualize it, but thank goodness, we caught him before he could finish.

Our child did not want to live.

We should have gone to a hospital, but that thought never crossed our minds. We went with what we knew.

We waited until he fell asleep. Ron and I talked. We argued and talked some more. I blamed him. He was so hard on Justin that this had to be his fault. I was digging my heels in because I knew gentle love and compassion were the answer, and I was angry. Fed up. This was it. Ron was wrong.

I began to think I might be better off without him.

CHAPTER 8

A Marriage on the Brink of Failure

We had a pointed conversation that night.

We knew we loved each other and that we were soulmates. But we also realized this situation was tearing us apart. Somehow, we had to get on the same page. But how could we do this? There were so many "But how?" questions.

We screamed and yelled for hours. Neither of us was listening to what the other said. We were getting nowhere.

Stefanye came in crying, begging us not to get a divorce. It was the punch in the gut that got us to calm down.

Neither of us wanted that.

We needed something to agree on. This was important.

I was too lenient; Ron was too tough. We could agree on this, and somehow, we understood that there was a place for both the toughness and the leniency. We could agree that we loved each other and our children above everything else.

We agreed we respected each other. I would have to toughen up and Ron would need to tone down, based on the needs of the situation. We knew that Justin tried to take his life twice and we had to face the fact that this problem was bigger than us. We vowed to each other that we were not going to grow apart and that no matter how hard things got, we would grow together.

This promise would be tested.

CHAPTER 9

Taking on the Monster

The next day, we made an appointment with our pediatrician because we trusted him above anyone else.

Suicide became a monster we needed to defeat.

We were ready to take on the monster.

Thus began the three-year long parade of doctors and misdiagnoses.

The monster would continue to attack us for another year.

Our pediatrician had been prescribing Justin's medications, but he suggested a psychiatrist might be a better option. He recommended someone, and we went and met with him.

I'll never forget the first (and only) appointment with this doctor. He had messy white hair. He looked like a mad scientist. He asked questions and said things that didn't make sense, but Ron and I were in such a place of vulnerability that we listened in silence.

Justin wasn't the only one losing confidence. We had no idea how to parent our child. Nothing was working, and we were open to anything that might help.

The doctor told us our child had to be on "suicide watch."

Suicide watch.

Seriously?

How?

What did this mean?

His advice was to put Justin on a high-potency drug called Risperdal—

it is a form of Haldol, a strong antidepressant.

The doctor also instructed us on how to restrain Justin so he wouldn't thrash around. The idea was that we had to keep him from hurting himself. And, of course, under no circumstances could he be alone.

Never alone.

How do you do that?

The most important thing became keeping Justin safe. We cleared out his room. Everything came out except for the mattress. He had no toys, no dresser, no sheets, nothing. Only a mattress.

We had to move knives and scissors to a high place where he could not easily get to them. Thankfully, he had not experienced any growth spurts yet, so he was not very tall!

Who would have thought that everyday things could become weapons for self-destruction?

Pens and pencils—daggers. Weapons.

But he needed pencils to do schoolwork.

Since he was never going to be left alone, we put them in places where we could get to him before he could get to them.

We had to do the same thing at school. He was not allowed to have anything in his desk. The teachers would loan him a pencil to do work and collect it when the assignment was complete.

Our lives were totally and completely upside down.

A happy day was rare.

We stayed so vigilant that my eyes hurt.

Although Stefanye and Konnor never said a word, we knew this impacted them. We didn't have the energy to talk with them about it. Much went unspoken. They were older now—Stefanye at age 17 was rarely home, and Konnor, at age 14, retreated to his room. We all did our best to cope.

Shortly after our meeting with the psychologist, a first few days into

Justin being on this hefty medication, it was time for the school's spring choir concert. Ron and I sat in the audience with our best "happy" masks on. We did this a lot.

We noticed that while Justin was onstage singing, he kept sticking out his tongue. The kids did a parade around the audience, and when he walked by us, we whispered to him to keep his tongue in his mouth. But of course, he didn't listen. When we got in the car to go home, we again told him to stop doing that thing with his tongue.

As was typical, he became defiant and insisted he wasn't doing anything with his tongue.

It was so relentless and so odd that Ron and I decided to believe him. If he couldn't control his tongue, then maybe something was wrong? I called our pediatrician. He told me this was a side effect of the medication and to get to the emergency room immediately.

Yikes!

Could anything go right?

He really couldn't control this. It turned out the medication was causing his tongue to swell. If we had let him go to sleep, he would have suffocated.

The ER doctors gave Justin epinephrine to stop the swelling, watched him for a while, and sent us home.

Just another day in the Bachman household.

We decided our time with the psychiatrist was over.

We tried another doctor, who suggested Justin might have Asperger's or perhaps he was on the Autism spectrum. There was a pediatrician who specialized in working with Autistic kids, so we made an appointment.

Ron and I decided we would talk with this doctor first, meet him, and review the history before bringing Justin to see him. We went during the school day so Justin would not have to be left alone.

The new doctor's office was in a wealthy part of town. I worked from home, so I tended to dress casually, and Ron, being in home repair, was always dressed in messy clothes that were covered in paint, caulk, or stained with something.

This doctor came into the room where we were waiting and looked down his nose at us. It was so obvious, I almost laughed. He was arrogant and rude, and he made everything sound like our fault. I was stoic during the appointment, but when I got three steps out of the office I burst into tears. I told Ron I would never set foot in that office again.

We had hit another dead end in the maze that was our life. We had to find another path.

We returned to Cleveland Clinic for more evaluations. They diagnosed Justin with oppositional defiance disorder. Another label with no action.

Nobody was helping us.

Nobody was telling us what to do.

How should we be raising this child who had so many behavioral challenges?

The storms were not subsiding. We now knew how to restrain him, but all that did was leave us with bruises.

The Bachman Zombies marched onward.

We got the name of another doctor who was the head of the department of psychology at the Cleveland Clinic. We figured if he was the head of the department, he must be good.

Ron and I met with him a few times, and then we scheduled a session with Justin. At one point, the doctor sat back in his chair, as if he were having an epiphany. He looked at Justin and asked, "Justin, do you hear voices?"

"Yes, all the time."

"Do the voices make you do things?"

"Yes, they do," he said, with a facial expression like, "Duh! Of course."

"Justin, can you sit with the nurse in the waiting room so I can talk with your parents?"

Justin stepped out, and the doctor looked at us with the most serious expression and said, "I believe Justin is dealing with paranoid schizophrenia."

No way.

Our son is not schizophrenic.

Absolutely not.

This guy is off his rocker.

At this point, we were so desperate—but not desperate enough to believe this. There was no way our son was being driven by the voice of the devil—which was what we incorrectly understood psychosis to be.

We walked into the waiting room and looked at Justin.

I said, "Justin, the doctor asked you if you were hearing voices, and you answered yes. Can you explain why you answered yes?"

"Well, I hear your voice and Dad's voice and Stef's voice and Konnor's voice, my teacher's voice—"

We cut him off, or he would have continued to list all the voices he heard. I asked him if he had voices inside his head telling him to do bad things?

He looked at me like I was crazy.

Chalk up another bad diagnosis—another doctor searching so hard for labels, he couldn't see our kid.

What next?

We didn't have a lot of people to turn to.

I made an appointment with my psychologist. Dr. D was helpful, but I only let her in so far. My fear held me back.

With Justin on suicide watch and no indication this watch would be coming to an end soon, our friends started to disappear—or should I say, people we assumed were our friends went away.

Fortunately, Stefanye had one friend in particular, Star, who was always there for her. Star knew what was happening, and although Stef often stayed at her house, Star spent time at ours too. She wasn't afraid of Justin, and we were so thankful for her. Stefanye had her driver's license by then, so she had some flexibility. She was not unaffected—in fact, she was absolutely impacted, but she had the outlet of her social life to mitigate things.

She also had her guidance counselor at school. Mrs. Dingman was the most wonderful outlet for Stef. Mrs. Dingman would call us to keep us updated on Stefanye's mindset. It helped Ron and me to be more aware of how this was impacting our daughter—she was a Godsend, a little shining light in the darkness.

Konnor was a different story. He had a social group of six boys who were so close we called them the Magnificent Seven. They met in first grade and had remained friends over the years. At this point, they were in the seventh grade. When the boys started hanging out, Ron and I got to know the parents, and we began socializing with them and bringing everyone together. We were together a lot—some kind of dinner or activity almost every weekend. Because I worked from home, and because we lived within walking distance of our city recreation center, the boys were always at our house. Always. I loved it! They were great kids, and I was thrilled that Konnor had such a wonderful group of friends. We all assumed they would be friends for life.

Unfortunately, as Justin's challenges increased, the friends came around less and less.

We learned they did things without including us. I processed this with my therapist, and she pointed out that we had been so secretive about what was happening with Justin, maybe they were fearful. She suggested I let them in. How could they help if they didn't understand?

Since I felt these were my closest friends, it made sense to invite them into my experience. So, I scheduled one-on-one coffee dates with four of them. I explained what was happening with Justin, and I even told them he had attempted suicide and was on "suicide watch." I explained that this meant we could not leave him alone.

I allowed myself to be vulnerable.

I used the "S" word.

I prayed they would understand. All I wanted was a hug and a friend.

The first person I had coffee with called me a helicopter parent—a hoverer. I was stunned that she would say such a thing. She said that Justin was far too young to really be able to know what he was doing—that if we loosened up and left him alone, he would be fine. I went on to explain that the doctors told us to stay with him, and I asked her to please continue to include us and to please understand when we couldn't join in. I emphasized that I especially wanted to be included in girls' nights because Ron could be with Justin. We left with the promise that I would be.

Shortly after that conversation, I heard there was a girls' night, but no one called me.

I was devastated.

The next meeting was not much better. This person told me we were really not that close, and were more like "Hi, how are you friends." This made no sense to me whatsoever. We had gone out socially and done things as families for *years*. She had confided in me. How could she say this? Shortly after our coffee date, her husband called and suggested we get Justin "A few sessions with a psychologist and he would be fine."

Nope—been there, done that.

The third and fourth friends were more empathetic and asked a lot of questions, but in the end, they stopped calling too. Their boys stopped coming over, and they stopped including Konnor in anything. Although Konnor never complained, I know he was hurt.

We were alone. I have never felt more isolated.

Not only did Justin not have friends, now we didn't either.

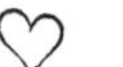  

Things were bad at the start of Justin's fourth-grade year. He was deeply depressed and never out of our sight unless he was asleep. Ron or I drove him to and from school and walked him to the door, where he was greeted by a teacher.

This was the only concession the school was willing to make. Essentially, they penalized Justin. They refused to put him on an IEP, and they took away his recess. We asked for an aide to be with him on the playground, but the school refused.

Here was a kid with severe ADHD who had trouble sitting still, and their answer was to punish him—send him to the office to sit alone during recess.

More heartbreak.

The guidance counselor was no help. This was during the period that Justin was not allowed to have any sharp objects. We found out that the counselor would occasionally invite Justin into his office to throw darts at his dartboard. You might think, "Oh, they must have been Velcro." Nope, the real sharp, pointy darts. The guidance counselor gave our child—*our child who wanted to harm himself*—dangerously sharp objects.

This was one of three instances during Justin's school years when I became a stark raving lunatic. I laid into this counselor and asked him what the hell he was thinking. This was a kid who had to borrow a pencil from a teacher, and he was giving him darts? I went bonkers, but there wasn't much I could do. He was the only guidance counselor in the school. I made it clear that this was never to happen again.

We really liked Justin's fourth-grade teacher, Mrs. Chonko. She had taught Konnor, and she was willing to work with us. She did the best she could to advocate for extra services for Justin but the Principal provided zero support.

On October 3, almost one year after Justin's first suicide attempt, my phone rang.

I answered.

It was the school secretary. "Get here right away, your son is trying to kill himself."

I don't remember much about what happened next. I shifted into autopilot. Somehow, I got into my car and drove to school, but I can't tell you what route I took or if I stopped at red lights. I didn't even know where I parked.

When I arrived, I saw police cars, and I ran inside. There was someone waiting for me at the door. I have no idea who that person was, but I remember them saying "Gym," and I took off running.

Someone was talking, explaining what had happened. It was hard to listen.

I was told the kids had been in the gym with a substitute teacher. Awful sign number one. *Shit.*

The kids were told to pick partners and, of course, one student had to be with Justin. Unfortunately, the child made a stink about not wanting to be paired with him.

Boom.

Lightning.

Thunder.

This was a hurricane.

The ensuing storm was like nothing anyone at school had ever seen. Justin started screaming and yelling: "No one wants to be my partner because I'm worthless! I'll make this easy and kill myself."

The bleachers in the gym were pushed back against the wall. I'm told he climbed up to the top and announced to whoever would listen he was going to dive headfirst onto the gym floor to die.

Someone immediately rushed the students out of the gym, and someone else ran for Justin's classroom teacher, Mrs. Chonko. She grabbed him and held him until I got there. Her arms were bruised because he struggled hard to get out of her grasp so he could finally make this thing happen—hence the reason the police were called.

This all occurred quickly. By the time I got to the gym, Justin wasn't there, and I was ushered into a room nearby. I begged for my son. I screamed and insisted they get him for me.

I was so afraid he would be arrested.

My memory of these moments is scattered. My brain is still protecting me. I knew I didn't want anyone taking my child away from us. I knew the police were there, and I had this awful, gut-wrenching feeling he was being interrogated or maybe someone was trying to help—but I firmly believed nobody outside of our family could.

I believed Ron and I could deal with it. It was our problem, our job.

Finally they brought Justin to me. Someone talked to me—I don't know who it was—but they suggested I take Justin to the hospital.

I refused.

I could handle this.

This person said, "Your son attempted suicide and needs help."

I knew that. They didn't have to remind me.

In hindsight, I should have let them take him to the hospital. It's what I recommend now.

The compromise was that we call the psychologist to tell her what had happened. They let me take Justin under the condition we would go straight to her office. I agreed, and that is what I did.

Ron met us there. The psychologist didn't give us a choice. She said she had already called the hospital and was having Justin admitted.

There was no more hiding.

We had to hospitalize our son.

CHAPTER 10

Trapped

The day we took Justin to the hospital—the day he was admitted to the mental ward for attempted suicide—was the hardest day of our lives.

Of course, they didn't call it the "mental ward," but that was how we saw it.

The looney bin.

The place for crazy people.

But our son wasn't crazy.

He wasn't.

It felt like a tsunami had rolled in, knocked us off our feet, and swept us away. We had no choice—well, we did have a choice. We could have continued to do the things we had been doing. But clearly, that was not working.

We had to face it. Something incomprehensible: Our child really and truly didn't want to live.

He believes death is the answer.

We didn't understand it. How could a child so beautiful and smart, a child who had beaten the 98% odds against him as an infant, not want to live?

He was loved.

It wasn't enough.

He needed his pain to go away.

He craved an escape. The only solution he saw was ending his life.

Justin loved us. In fact, he loved us so much, he believed his death would relieve us. He knew he was a difficult child and believed we didn't deserve to have our lives ruined because of him.

How fucking twisted is that?

I felt I had failed at the most important job of my life—being a parent. I had three chances. I did okay with the first two—Stef and Konnor—but not this child.

How could I continue parenting three children when one needed so much more than the others?

I was supposed to know how to juggle, but I didn't.

In that moment, my job was keeping Justin alive.

A huge decision loomed in front of us. We had been going to doctors for years and still had no answers. We had a monumental responsibility for our son's psyche—his mental health—and this was terrifying. We could no longer handle him, nor could we keep him safe. We were going to have to admit him to the hospital.

That realization tore my guts out.

Looking back, I know this was not a failure. But that day, I felt I had failed miserably at the most important job of my life.

CHAPTER 11

The Doors Closed Behind Us

When we got to the hospital, I figured we would get Justin settled and then Ron would go home and get me some things because I would stay, like I did when Justin was a baby.

The doctor came out to talk with us. He talked and he kept talking, but I heard only one thing. His words knocked every bit of wind out of my lungs.

I was not allowed to stay.

This had never occurred to me. How could this be? We had never left Justin overnight.

I argued with the doctor.

How can I leave my child alone? He is only ten years old.

The doctor held his ground. He was nice and kind, but he wasn't giving in.

Hospital policy.

Screw hospital policy!

Nope, we had to leave.

How could we?

I was ready to camp out in the waiting room.

I can close my eyes and vividly remember this scene. It plays out in my head like I was outside of my body. This couldn't be happening.

Ron and I were sitting in this small waiting room and Justin was standing next to us. There was a nurse, and the doctor was talking again.

Didn't he know I didn't want to hear any of this? Inside my head, I was screaming "Shut up!" but the words would not come out.

My world was shattering into a million tiny pieces of glass.

In the next moment, Justin moved and stood between Ron and me. He put his small hands on our shoulders, and put his face close to ours, and in a whisper that was barely audible, he said, "It's okay, Mom and Dad. I'm going to go in, and I'm going to come out a new Justin."

Tears started in the tips of our toes and came out with such force.

Choking sobs.

We were crying as if we were in mourning, as if someone had died.

Justin was telling us he needed help. He wanted help.

We had to give it to him.

This beautiful child we loved with our hearts and souls needed us to give this to him.

The doctor took him by the hand, and they walked down the short hall through the double doors. Justin never turned back. He was doing what he needed to do.

Slowly, the doors closed.

Our son was behind locked doors. He was a patient in a mental health facility.

I can still feel those doors closing. In fact, to this day, when I see doors like that, I react. Even if it's in a television show, I still cry.

Nobody should ever have to feel the despair Ron and I felt in that moment. Nobody.

We were told we could visit Justin for thirty minutes a day. If we were late, our time would be shortened. There was no need to worry about that, we would be there. I would arrive an hour early.

Ron and I sat in that waiting room for a while. I have no idea how long. We were numb. The clock didn't exist. We didn't know what to think, we didn't know what to do. We held each other tight and sobbed. To this day, I don't think I've ever cried that hard or felt so helpless. Even though we were going through it as a family, we were all alone.

CHAPTER 12

Riding the Roller Coaster of Guilt

I didn't know if we were doing the right thing. That made it harder. How could being separated from our child possibly be the right thing?

To make matters worse, we had to go home and tell our other two kids. Because this attempt was so public, we had no idea what anyone knew or what people were saying. Did everyone know? We were in such a state that the judgments of others didn't seem important.

Telling Stefanye and Konnor sucked.

Here's another thing the parenting books don't teach you. We had no idea how to do this. So, we sat them down and told them what happened in the gym. They knew how Justin reacted, so that part was not a surprise. The thing that stunned them both, and even stunned Ron and me, was using the words: *attempted suicide.*

We had not said this to them before, but they knew. Konnor was in eighth grade, and Stefanye was in eleventh, so they absolutely understood what was happening. But hearing the word and associating it with your own brother, or son, is beyond anything I can describe.

Of course, Stefanye and Konnor were worried. They wanted to know how long Justin would be away and what was happening to him. They wanted to visit, but only Ron and I were allowed.

We sat together as a family, minus one, and we cried.

There were so many things running through our heads. I feared this was harder on Stef and Konnor because they had to go to school the next day with no idea what they would be facing.

Would other kids even know? If they did, would they treat them differently?

We were honest with them. They asked us what to say, and we said we didn't know. Looking back, it wasn't helpful, but it was the best we could do. We told them to do what they felt was right in their hearts. They were under no obligation to explain anything to anyone.

So many people in our community—schools, sport teams, synagogue, work—knew. But nobody called.

Nobody.

Our house simply became a quiet place. None of us did much talking. We were all trying to process this in our own way. Each of us was wrapped up in our own fear, but we were together. Quiet, but together. There wasn't anything to say. And that had to be okay.

I'm not sure how we got through. It felt like we were operating on autopilot, but at the same time, we had to try to remember to do things—like eat. We didn't cook. We had no energy. Shopping—that didn't happen. Ron and I tried to go to Walmart because we knew we needed groceries. We went with no list, and I have no recollection if we walked out with anything resembling a nutritious meal, but I do remember feeling relieved we didn't bump into anyone we knew.

In a situation where someone is hospitalized for an injury or is going through cancer treatment, the meal trains line up and people bring food and stop by to offer support. This doesn't happen with mental illness.

This didn't happen for us. There were no friends lining up to do anything.

We were on our own.

We could barely say the word suicide. We were so afraid of the judgment of others, and for good reason. The judges, juries, and executioners were lining up with all their reasons why this was our fault.

We hovered too much.

We let him get away with bad behavior.

Find a good shrink, and he will be fine.

These are the things "well-meaning" people said to us.

After a few days, one of the girls in our old friend group—the magnificent seven of boys Konnor's age—called because she heard about what happened at school and "that Justin was in a program." Although it was nice, it didn't seem real to me. She had not called in months, and not only had she socially excluded Ron and me, her kids excluded Konnor.

It was all too easy for me to deflect my anger at the entire situation onto her. Sadly, my immediate thought was that her call was gossip oriented, because she wanted to know what really happened. She wanted to know if Justin was really "hospitalized." To this day, I have no idea if my assumption was right or wrong, but to me, it felt like she was looking for gossip.

I went into self-protection mode.

I was straight with her and thanked her for calling but said I had more on my plate than I could handle and talking about what happened was not something I was prepared to do. I told her that if she truly wanted to be friends, then it would have to be her actions that did the talking. I told her help would be appreciated. Could she send a meal?

I never heard from her again.

Motive confirmed—or was it?

Hindsight has given me insight. Maybe she did call to gossip, but she may also have been afraid. No one knew what to say. *We* didn't. Grace and compassion were needed on all sides, but the enormity of the situation blinded me. I wanted people to set aside their fears to show me compassion, but I didn't know how to ask for it. I had no capacity to recognize how scary it was for someone to try to talk with me. I built a giant wall and kept everyone on the other side.

I longed for that friend who realized I was grieving. I needed someone to be judgment free, to give me the grace to feel what I was feeling without offering suggestions. There was no solution, and I needed someone to acknowledge my pain and tell me they cared. I needed someone to look past the bad energy I was putting forward because the real me, the one who was so afraid, was in there. The vulnerable me was under that defensive layer. I needed someone to look beneath the surface I showed on the outside.

I needed so much. And I didn't know how to ask for it.

We took our half-hour-a-day visit with Justin seriously. We never missed it, and we were comforted by the fact that Justin seemed okay. He was happy to see us and that felt good.

I got my butterfly kisses and that meant the world.

After Justin was there for a week, we had our first formal meeting with the in-patient doctor. We liked him right away. Dr. S told us that he noticed Justin was fidgety and could not sit still. He felt Justin would do better on a higher dose of medication and he needed our permission to increase Justin's Ritalin from 10 mg to 40 mg.

This seemed like a huge jump, and it scared the daylights out of us, but the doctor explained that he was in a safe environment for a trial.

We agreed. We were desperate, we would try whatever would help our son.

At the end of the second week, we met with Dr. S again, and he said there was a marked improvement in Justin's behavior. The increased dose of Ritalin was working. He told us that in a few days, he could leave the hospital.

I should have been overjoyed. Our son was coming home from the hospital! But he was safe there and our house was peaceful. I hated myself for feeling that way, but it had been a relief not to fear the possibility of a storm or—God forbid—another suicide attempt.

I rode on a rollercoaster of guilt.

Were we equipped to deal with him?

Would the increase in medication mean no more storms?

Was he cured?

Did he still want to take his life?

Maybe he wasn't feeling worthless in this moment, but what would happen once he was back in the old routine?

Could I ask Konnor not to be a regular big brother? To not piss Justin off? Could we ask everyone to behave perfectly and not do anything that could possibly upset Justin? Absolutely not. This wasn't going to happen, so how were we supposed to live?

There were no answers.

Clearly, Justin was still on suicide watch, but when could he come off it?

Thankfully, the doctors had a follow-on, in-home care solution. This meant there would be an outpatient counselor who would work with Justin in our home.

When we finally got home, there was no celebration. After the meningitis, we were so happy and felt like we had left the illness behind.

Not this time. Our son was still sick, but with something no one could see or understand. The demons had not left the building.

Because we were still in somewhat of a zombie state, we didn't ask all the questions we needed to ask of Dr. S. It might seem obvious that we should have asked about Justin returning to school, but we didn't. We should have asked how to explain things to people who asked questions, but we didn't. We didn't ask about diet, activity, being around other people—so many things…but we didn't ask.

We needed answers and called the hospital and left a message for Dr. S. About an hour later, we got a call back from the head of the department—the one who incorrectly diagnosed Justin as a schizophrenic. We didn't want to talk with him, we wanted to speak with Dr. S. He knew Justin and had been treating him.

This doctor refused to let us talk with Dr. S, the one we trusted. We hung up and called back again. When leaving the message, I was specific. I told the nurse that we wanted a call back from Dr. S, not anyone else.

Imagine our surprise when the same doctor called us again and told us we were not permitted to talk with Dr. S.

I was dumbstruck. Both Ron and I, as well as Justin, had started a great relationship with Dr. S, but now we couldn't talk with him? It made no sense.

It was scary how few things made sense.

Justin came home on a Friday, and on Monday, the outpatient counselor came over. He was awful. I don't even remember his name. He was bland and boring. He spoke in a monotone, and it was obvious from the moment he walked into our home that this was not going to be a good (or even mediocre) fit.

The only thing he did was give us a note stating that Justin could return to school. We asked how to explain this to the school and his answer was "Do what is comfortable for you."

Really? Do what is comfortable? Nothing was comfortable. Nothing.

Someone was playing a cruel joke on us.

Our journey through the maze hit another wall; once again, we had to turn around and find a new path.

We knew Justin needed to go back to school.

We had called the principal the day after the suicide attempt to let her know Justin was in the hospital and would be absent for a few weeks. The principal had reassured us that they had handled the situation and had not used the word suicide. They told the students Justin was out sick. We listened without asking questions.

The following day, Justin showed up back at school.

This was a mistake. We should have gone and met with his teacher and the principal. We should have gotten more details about what happened that day and what they told the kids. We should have filled them in on the things the doctors told us about Justin's medication and how he was so much calmer now.

On his first day back, I dropped Justin off into the hands of the person at the door, and I went home. I watched the clock anxiously. I held my breath throughout the day and jumped whenever my phone rang. I was certain it would be school calling to send him home because something had happened. I felt pretty good when the clock hit 2:30 and it was time for me to pick Justin up. I assumed it must have been an okay day.

Wrong. As soon as he saw me, he burst into tears.

It was the same routine.

"I'm never going back."

"Every kid hates me."

"All the kids were mean."

But he added something to the mix. He said the kids were told he was gone for good because he had been expelled.

Expelled?

Shortly after I got Justin home, the phone rang. It was one of our neighbors, Sally, who had a child in Justin's grade—not his class, but the same grade. We had been friendly with the family, but the boys didn't really socialize—Justin didn't socialize with anyone.

I about fell out of my chair upon hearing her story of what happened at school.

There were other neighbors, the Topper family, whom we didn't like. They were the kind of people who always had to "top" what you were doing. Everything was always about them. Their son Lucien was Justin's age, and this kid had a history of tormenting Justin. He was the definition of a bully. We had ignored it, but I could not ignore this.

Sally told me Lucien started a rumor that Justin was expelled from school for attacking a teacher. Lucien had told so many kids that they were all surprised and frightened when Justin came back.

None of this made sense. Didn't the teachers hear about this rumor—something? Anything? I was so thankful to Sally for calling.

I was livid. How could this child be allowed to do this? I picked up the phone and called Mrs. Topper to talk with her, assuming her son would apologize and set things straight.

Wrong.

She called me a liar. She said her son would never do anything of the sort and told me I should focus on the problems in my home. She repeated that Lucien would never do such a thing, and she questioned my integrity for making such an accusation.

Where was the hidden camera? This could not be happening.

I had my child to worry about. I called Ron so he could come home and we could handle this together. We had to convince Justin he needed to go to school the next day. That would not be easy.

About an hour later, my phone rang, and it was the principal. She told me that Mrs. Topper had come to the school, in person, to tell her about our phone call. Mrs. Topper admitted Lucien started the rumor, but she made up another egregious lie.

She told the principal her middle child, Leon (who was in high school with both my older kids), would be having life-threatening (her exact words) surgery the next day, so could they please give her younger son a "pass"—because after all, what Justin did was far worse. The reason for the principal's call was to let me know they were simply going to "Let the situation go."

What?

I was beyond livid now.

I was spitting nails.

I didn't care for this principal, so I hung up. I didn't have the energy for an argument. I knew this kid was not having "life-threatening" surgery. My two older kids were not friends with Leon, but they had seen him in school every single day. How does a kid facing that kind of surgery behave like his normal self in school every day? Stefanye and

Konnor were beside themselves. They were ready to take this kid down.

We made them promise not to say anything. After all, the kid may not have known about his mother's lie.

The next morning, Ron and I made it a point to watch Leon get in his car and drive to school. I also watched for him to come home from school that same day—which he did, right on time. Unless he drove himself to the hospital, had surgery, and was home by 3:00, something was amiss. My older kids saw Leon at school that day and all the following days too. This woman made the entire thing up.

What could we do?

Absolutely nothing.

This would not be the last unfortunate interaction we would have with this family.

Three years later, Mrs. Topper called the middle school to speak with the assistant principal. She told him that Justin punched Lucien on the bus ride home. What she failed to realize was that the assistant principal not only knew that Justin never rode the bus, but that Justin was at an afterschool event. There was no way this complaint could be true. She had blatantly lied again. But score one for the good guys—she got busted!

Dealing with these neighbors was one of the biggest lessons we learned through this wild journey. As a family, we sat down and talked about what Ron named "controlling the controllable." We could not control anything this neighbor from hell said or did, but we could control our actions and our responses—and behave morally, even if other people didn't. Together, we decided that if we made a big deal out of this, the Toppers would find a way to make it about them. We had no idea how they would behave, so we opted to do nothing and deprive them of any satisfaction.

Justin returned to school, and the storm clouds began to cluster again. We heard thunderclaps in the distance, but this time, the wind was changing. Mary Poppins opened her trusty umbrella and floated down into our lives.

———

CHAPTER 13

Finding Mary Poppins

As bad as the Topper family was, that's how great our next-door neighbors were. We bonded with them the day we moved to this neighborhood and although they didn't know what went on behind our closed doors, they had been wonderful family friends for more than six years. They had two children, the same ages as Stefanye and Konnor, who lived with a medical condition called Fragile X. Although different from autism, the characteristics look similar. Neither child had language, but that didn't matter to our kids. About a month after Justin came home from the hospital, the parents came to tell us they were joining a special-needs baseball league and asked if our kids would be their partners. We were thrilled and immediately agreed.

At a game, we met another family who told us about their friend from law school. After graduation, this friend decided law wasn't for her, and she went back for her degree in social work. She had recently returned to Cleveland and started a practice, visiting people's homes to provide counseling. She wasn't a psychologist, but she was a licensed social worker.

I got her number and called immediately. We had a fantastic phone conversation and scheduled our first visit. We didn't know it yet, but this was the spoonful of sugar we needed to make the medicine go down.

I was beside myself with dread the first time she came over. Justin wanted no part of her. He was in fine Justin form—yelling, screaming, and being particularly obstinate. Thinking Mary was about to flee the building, I gave him an ultimatum under my breath. "Get downstairs, or there will be serious consequences." This didn't work, and instead, a full-fledged storm rolled in.

Justin shouted that we could not force him to talk with someone he didn't want to talk with. He slammed the door to his room and yelled that we could not make him come out. He called us names, like mean and dumb.

I was so embarrassed I wanted to crawl into a hole. I could barely look this woman in the eye. But she was so kind and understanding and said this was just the thing she needed to see. She didn't judge us. She empathized, and then, she took charge.

Mary walked up the stairs and sat on the floor outside of Justin's room. Through the door, she told Justin she was excited to meet him. When he yelled, she stopped talking and waited for him to be quiet. The louder he got, the quieter she spoke. This essentially forced him to listen to her.

After a while, she opened his bedroom door, sat cross-legged on the floor, smiled, and told Justin she would be happy to wait until he was calm and ready.

And she waited.

She sat there and didn't say a word. She just waited.

She didn't react to anything he did or said.

I was distraught, wondering how long she would be willing to sit there. She had no clue how bullheaded our son could be. I was certain she would give up and never come back.

Justin did his typical thing and stomped around. He didn't have anything to throw because we had taken everything out of the room. He jumped, lay on the floor, kicked, and screamed.

None of this got a rise out of Mary. She continued to sit patiently and wait.

After what felt like hours (it was probably about thirty minutes),

Justin moved to the doorway and sat down in front of her with a scowl on his face. He even growled at her! The evil fingers popped out.

Then, she just started chatting with him as if nothing had happened. She began trying to figure out the things that interested him:

"What is your favorite sport?"

"What foods do you like to eat?"

At first, his answers were short, one-word grunts. But he slowly warmed up and gave her answers that were funny and made her laugh. Eventually, they were having a simple conversation. After about fifteen minutes of chatter, Mary thanked Justin for talking with her and asked him if they could talk again another time. He said, "Sure," and returned to whatever he had been doing before she arrived.

This was pure brilliance. She didn't feel like a doctor or a teacher to Justin.

She communicated with him.

She didn't ask him dumb questions like, "How do you feel?"

She earned his trust.

Remarkable.

This was a victory!

After that, Mary spent a little over an hour with Ron and me, explaining how she worked. The first thing she said was that she could help us, but only if we were willing to do hard things. She talked about consistency, and she told us we would need to be *really* tough, but if we were, Justin would get better.

We agreed.

Before she left, she wanted to do one thing, and she called Justin back to join us.

Thankfully, he willingly came into the room.

She told Justin that she was a lawyer and that lawyers made contracts. Justin was ten years old, but she did a great job of explaining that when you sign a contract, you are bound to its terms. She handwrote a contract that said Justin was not allowed to hurt himself and that if he felt like he needed to hurt himself, he would tell Mom and Dad first, before he did anything.

We all signed the document, and to this day he has abided by that agreement.

This wasn't a magic bullet. There were a few instances when we had to remind him of the agreement, but he held to it.

Mary came to our house two or three days each week, and she stayed for hours—sometimes two and as many as four or five. She stayed as long as was needed.

Unfortunately, insurance did not cover her services, and she was not cheap, but she was worth every penny we spent. We struggled financially for many years. We even took out a second mortgage. Unfortunately, we also had to dip into the kids' college funds, but we did what we needed to do. It was humbling to apply for hardship tuition when Stefanye went off to college, and it has taken us more than ten years to recover financially, but we would spend it again in a heartbeat. It was so worth it to save our son.

The first thing Mary did was talk with us about school. She let us know that the school sending Justin home was illegal and that we had the right for him to be on an IEP (Individualized Education Plan). The suicide attempt had convinced the administration that this was the case, so there was no argument. However, there was still a vast divide between what Justin needed and what the school was willing to provide.

She coached us on approaching the administration for a meeting and who should attend. She said she would be right there by our side during the meeting. Mary coached me on how to run the meeting and suggested I kick it off by talking about helping Justin succeed. I was friendly and upbeat, but I was firm in my intention that the school needed to step up. This was a kid with severe ADHD who had not been allowed to go to recess for the past two years. We demanded the school provide Justin with an aide who could help him navigate the playground.

We requested that a safe space be made where Justin could go when he felt stressed.

We requested all the typical things for a student with attention problems, including teacher notes and extended time for homework and tests.

We indicated we did not need the school psychologist's services because we had hired our own.

Most important, we told the school they could no longer send Justin home for what they deemed bad behavior. We pointed out that this was illegal and advised that if they attempted to send him home, we would not come to pick him up.

The school was not happy with any of our requests and rejected almost everything.

As I listened to their denials, I could feel my stress level rising, but Mary shot me looks that said, "Stay calm." An explosion on my part would not help.

They agreed to create a crisis plan. They had no choice on that point because they could not risk a suicide happening in school. They realized how close they had come to a horrifying tragedy. It was baffling that they didn't have a plan in place for students who escalated in behavior. Many people believe that children under the age of thirteen are too young for mental health issues as severe as suicide. Sadly, it is a fact, and schools are still not prepared. According to WebMD, suicide attempts in kids ages ten to twelve quadrupled between 2000 and 2020.

Against the wishes of the school, we asked Mary to write a crisis plan. She taught Justin's teacher how to recognize his behavior escalations and how to escort him out of the classroom before things got heated. She gave the school a blueprint for creating a small space in the PT (Physical Therapy) room. This space would have some soft pillows and blankets and be blocked off with partitions. It was available for use by any student, which was wonderful! We knew Justin would use it. We introduced this space to him when he was in a calm mood and let him know he was allowed to ask to go there whenever he felt he was getting out of control. But we also let him know this was not a free pass to get out of class.

Sadly, the school flat-out refused to provide Justin with help to participate in recess. They indicated that if he continued to have poor behavior, they would send him home. They also told us Mary was not welcome at the meetings. Mary, Ron, and I were all shocked that they could be so harsh and unbending. At one point, the principal stood up and yelled at us for being unreasonable. The meeting was a disaster.

Afterward, we sat down with Mary, who suggested we reach out to an attorney. It was the only way we would be able to make progress. She recommended someone she knew, and off we went to get legal assistance.

I'll never forget our first meeting in the attorney's office. Justin—my loud, talkative child—went mute. He refused to speak, then he put his head in the chair and told her to talk to his butt. It sounds funny, and she laughed, but Ron and I were mortified!

Thankfully, this attorney had a great reputation and a huge track record for success with the schools. She called a meeting, but the school put it off until the very last day required by law.

We quickly realized that the tactic this administration was using was to delay things as much as possible. Fourth grade was the last year Justin would be in their building, so they knew they could delay to the point where he would no longer be their problem. Unfortunately, they succeeded, and there was nothing we could do.

CHAPTER 14

Caring Teachers Make A Difference

Once we realized what the school was doing, our attorney suggested we meet with the principal of the middle school Justin would attend for fifth and sixth grade. She recommended we save our money and not have her attend, and see how things went without her.

Ron, Mary, and I called this meeting before fourth grade ended. We got another gift.

The middle school principal and his team turned out to be the complete opposite of everyone at the elementary school. The principal was kind and listened; together, the team made a real effort to figure out how to make things work. They were shocked that Justin had been denied recess, and they agreed that they would have team members alternate to ensure he would get some fresh air and activity every day.

The students in fifth grade had a team of three teachers, and we got the dream team, which included a wonderful interventionist. Over the summer, these amazing teachers worked with Mary and me to put together a plan that provided Justin with everything he needed.

Structure and consistency were critical. Mary pointed out that Justin had limited capacity to deal with surprises in his schedule. He didn't have the social wherewithal to adapt to changes, so we proactively began writing plans.

When school started, the interventionist wrote a schedule for Justin every day and would sit down with him to review it. This eliminated surprises and made sure they kept him on track. The administration called me if one of the teachers wouldn't be in school, so Justin would know to expect something different. The team of teachers was consistent, communicated with me, and did everything they said they would do. Every day.

It was amazing. Justin soared academically.

We did the exact same thing at home. We created lists that covered his day from the moment he woke up until he went to bed. They were extensive and detailed. There were no breaks for the weekend—this was a daily thing. These lists laid out Justin's responsibilities. For example, when he woke up, he brushed his teeth and ate breakfast. What he ate for breakfast was his choice, but we outlined the timing. I detailed an after-school schedule, so he knew my plan. If I had to run an errand, it was on the plan. In the past, doing something he didn't want to do would cause a storm, but because he was still on suicide watch, he could not be alone and would have to go with me. Mary explained that his reaction was a natural consequence to the unexpected activities.

These lists served multiple purposes. First, they provided structure. No surprises. If Justin didn't want to go to the store or brush his teeth, the lists allowed him to settle himself and accept the situation. If Justin tried to argue, my job was to point out that it was on the list and not engage. Similar to Mary's sitting on the floor waiting for Justin, I had to ignore the pushback and wait for him to calm down. If he caused me to be late, I was to point out that there would be consequences—but that was it! I was not allowed to argue or say anything.

This sounds simple, but it's really hard. Try ignoring a screaming kid—it drained every ounce of energy we had. But we stuck with it. This gave Justin a sense that he could achieve something. He knew if he stuck to the plan and there were no arguments, he would get better—a genuine incentive.

This was hard for all of us, because it took away any kind of spontaneity. We had to plan everything. We went about this for a few months. The first few weeks were filled with failures, better known as "First Attempt In Learning." This was learning we needed to do. We were adjusting to the process.

Justin was great at testing the limits. As a result, "No empty threats!" became our mantra. If cleaning his room was on the schedule and he wanted to play outside, he couldn't go until his room was clean. This was particularly hard for me. I was a softie, and I wanted him to be able to do the things he wanted to do; however, that was a big cause of our problems.

The more we held firm, the more Justin got it. But make no mistake, the consistency thing is rough. Really rough.

After about six months, Justin began having success. We still had a long way to go, but our house was so much more peaceful. The arguments were diminishing. A victory!

After Justin achieved one entire month of staying on schedule, without storms, we added in small amounts of unplanned time. For example, he could earn thirty minutes to do something of his choosing—it had to be approved, but he could choose. Most often, he chose video games.

After about a year, we loosened up on the scheduling and Justin started to own more of it. His sixth-grade teachers applied the schedule, and we used a looser version at home. They still always called when there was a substitute teacher or a fire drill, but the rigidity and detail became less necessary. When he entered seventh grade, Justin was able to use the agenda system used by all the students.

Although the structure and consistency of the schedules eliminated some triggers, Justin's personality was still explosive, and he had to learn how to calm down when things escalated. More important, Mary helped us realize when the storm was coming, and how to handle Justin before he got out of control.

We learned the technique she called "take ten."

We talked with Justin about this concept during a calm period, when there was no anger. It seemed so obvious, but with everything we had been through, there was no such thing as obvious!

Mary facilitated a discussion where we all talked about how we felt during the storms. We explained to Justin how afraid we were during these fits of rage and how much his actions and words hurt. He too hated the storms. Clearly, he did not like being so out of control.

We laid out a plan.

Mary told Justin that if Ron or I noticed he was starting to get upset, we would use a code phrase, "Take ten." This meant that Justin was to go into his room, and he had to stay there for ten minutes to calm down. We would set a timer. If he left his room before the ten minutes were up, the timer would start again.

Mary explained to Ron and me that we had to ignore his rage. We did not deserve to be spoken to in a disrespectful way, so we shouldn't listen.

If Justin refused to go into his room, we would turn our backs on him and not speak. We "took ten" until he calmed down. The idea was that life would not return to normal until he could control his behavior.

This sounded good in theory. Implementing the strategy in the heat of the moment was another story. Try ignoring a raving child who is pressing every single one of your buttons. It was just short of impossible.

Initially, Justin refused to go into his room. A part of me knew that he had to test us. He had to see how this would play out and what he could get away with. But the other part of me knew that these rages left him so out of control that he couldn't listen to what I was saying.

It was so easy for me to get mad *because* he was mad. I had a way of taking on his anger. I wasn't angry at the same thing, but I was angry that he was escalating. I knew this was going to inconvenience and impact my day in a negative way, so subconsciously, I was escalating almost as fast as he was. I learned that as the adult, I had to stay calm. I couldn't take on his problem and let it overtake me.

Again, great in theory, really rough in practice.

It took everything I had to be silent. The first time this happened, I lasted a few minutes. I quietly said, "Justin, you need to take ten." He might as well have flipped me the bird.

He continued yelling about how stupid I was and that he was mad. I turned my back, but he grabbed me and yelled that I needed to look at him. My immediate reaction was "This is nuts" and my repeating "Take ten" was never going to work. The more he yelled, the harder it was to stay quiet. After about five minutes, I turned around and yelled "Shut up and go take ten" at the top of my lungs. That stunned Justin into silence—for about a second—then the storm raged on.

I was defeated.

Now I was feeling sorry for myself. How could I ever be able to do this?

Mary kept encouraging us to be strong. She impressed upon us that the magic was in the consistency. We *had* to be consistent. We had to keep doing it. Keep trying. No giving up.

As time went on, we got better at ignoring the bad behavior and slowly (very slowly) but surely, with the work he was doing with Mary, and our consistency, Justin eventually learned to retreat to his room for ten minutes to calm himself.

When I say eventually, I mean it. This work took time. There was no fast solution.

Mary also practiced calming techniques with Justin on a regular basis. These were the tools he was to use when he was in his room taking ten, or at any moment when he felt his temper rising.

Mary did an exercise with Justin where he turned and walked away. Our kitchen was galley style with an eight-foot-long island. Justin would stand with Mary, and he would practice turning around and slowly walking to the other end of the kitchen. He was supposed to take deep breaths and count as he walked. She taught him to focus on the counting, breathing, and walking instead of his anger. He was learning to distract his mind from the anger to calm himself down.

This worked too, but it took practice and discipline. The walks were to be practiced daily. And it could not be "one and done." The only way to form a habit was to do it again and again and again—oh, and again!

The saying "practice makes perfect" is so true. It sounds odd, but calming himself down was a skill Justin needed to learn, and these were powerful tools. Calm periods were the best time to practice because muscle memory works.

When the anger did come—which was normal—Justin had to learn to deescalate himself. Mary knew Justin liked baseball and he had used a bat to hit things during many of his fits of rage. She suggested we turn this into a positive and purchase something called a "hit away"—an inexpensive piece of equipment baseball players use to practice batting. We got one and put it on one of the poles in our basement, and when Justin needed to blow off steam, he could productively swing the bat.

It didn't work at first, and it didn't work the second or third times either. But eventually, something kicked in. We had to remind Justin to use his tools, and when he was able to do so, the relief came.

The storms were diminishing. It was working. And then, a year later, and our house was calm, and the storms had passed.

However, there was more work to be done. Much more work.

CHAPTER 15

Distorted Thinking and Choosing Our Words Carefully

One day, Justin came home with a test marked 100%—a perfect score. I looked at it and said something like, "Wow! That's great! You got 100%, you are so smart."

His answer was, "No I'm not, it was easy," and the look I got was like I was the stupid one for not realizing *he* was the stupid one.

It sounds odd, but we didn't know how to talk with Justin. Mary explained that we had to learn a whole new language because Justin was experiencing distorted thinking. His brain worked in a way that was literal, and he was not processing what we would see as logical. When he said he was stupid, he believed it, and he believed it to the point where he perceived our telling him otherwise as a lie.

We really wrestled with this, until one day, he came home with a story that helped me see the light.

The kids at school rotated lunch jobs in the cafeteria. This included trash pickup, collecting trays, wiping tables, and sweeping the floors. There was a girl in his class who had the job of sweeping on one particular day. She went to sweep under the table and the broom accidentally hit Justin's leg. Because of his distorted thinking, Justin assumed this girl didn't like him and hit him with the broom on purpose. He got mad and yelled at her and told a teacher that she hit him. He had distorted this tiny, accidental situation into "No one likes me."

Because of all Justin's issues and our need for vigilance, his teacher called me when anything happened. It was important for us to stay in communication. When Justin got home, I already knew the real story.

This is how the conversation went:

"Mom, my day was terrible. Katie purposely hit me with a broom because she thinks I'm an idiot."

"Justin, your teacher told me what happened. It was an accident."

"No, it wasn't. Katie hates me, and everyone laughed at me."

"She was doing her job and sweeping the floor, and the broom accidentally hit you."

Justin stomped his feet, swung his arms and yelled at the top of his lungs, *"It was not an accident! She hates me and I looked stupid! You think it is funny that everyone was laughing at me. I hate you! I hate you! You care more about her than me!"*

It only got worse from there. Luckily, Mary would arrive within the hour, and I knew we could process this with her.

Mary explained to us that Justin's thoughts, although wrong, were what he perceived to be the true way the incident occurred. He believed he got hit with the broom and that he was the cafeteria laughingstock. Mary suggested we not jump to conclusions even though we knew the truth. Our goal had to be to get Justin to come around to a point where he could reconsider the situation.

Mary helped us roleplay a better conversation, and then we invited Justin for another try.

She asked Justin what happened, and he said, "Katie purposely hit me with a broom today."

To which I replied, "Oh, my goodness, what happened?"

"I just told you, she hit me with the broom."

"Well, how did it happen? Did she swing it like a baseball bat?"

"No, Mom," he said, as he rolled his eyes. "I was sitting at the table, and she hit my feet. She doesn't like me, and the other kids were laughing. She thinks I'm an idiot."

I completely ignored the second part of his sentence and replied, "Hmm…was there garbage on the floor under the table?"

"I don't know. I doubt it."

"Well, let's think about this. Could it be possible that because she was cleaning up after lunch that maybe there was garbage under the table?"

"Maybe."

"Could it be possible there was garbage you didn't see, and she was doing her job of sweeping?"

"Maybe, but she still hit me."

"Could it be possible that maybe by accident, she didn't realize your feet were there?"

"No, Mom. She hates me, and she hit me on purpose."

"I know you are not friends, but just think about it. Could there be a small chance that it really was an accident?"

"Maybe."

"So what did you do, how did you handle it?"

"I told the teacher."

"Did you have a storm?"

"No."

"Great! I'm happy you didn't have a storm."

And that's where the conversation ended. We had to guide him to reconsider the assumptions he made. Mary taught us that at no point were we to agree or disagree, even when we knew what really happened.

I was coached to end the conversation with an "I" statement, noting my feelings. I could not say anything like, "You must be happy you didn't have a storm," because under no circumstances could I assume what he was thinking. I could have my thoughts, but I could not make assumptions about his. The trickiest part was not to validate or invalidate his thinking. He was entitled to his thoughts and feelings. We could not take that away from him. But we could not feed into something that wasn't right by engaging, and we certainly did not have to agree.

Ron and I were learning a whole new way to parent Justin.

Mary continued to help us adjust the way we spoke with Justin. When he came home with a good grade, or any kind of accomplishment, we had to use questions to work on creating conversations. Short, sweet conversations. At first, they looked something like this:

"Can you sign my test?

"I see you got 100%." Now I knew to just state the facts.

"Yeah, it was easy."

"I love it when things are easy!" I stated my opinion.

Short and sweet.

We had to be careful in choosing our words to ensure they didn't invoke something he could distort.

We also had to carefully ignore the parts of Justin's rhetoric that we knew he exaggerated. We were instructed not to feed into blanket statements, like, "No one likes me." This was tough because in the reality of that time, he didn't have friends. But none of this mattered. We simply had to steer his brain to consider more angles than the blanket statement. We had to get him to consider that his thinking might not be accurate.

This was complicated. Ron and I felt like we had to become experts at evaluating each situation to figure out what was real and what was blown out of proportion. We didn't want to make a mistake and minimize something that needed attention, but we couldn't further exacerbate a situation either.

Did I mention we were mentally exhausted?

Again, it came down to practice. We didn't always do it the right way, but when we did, we nailed it! Every victory paved the way for the future.

These discussions permeated our daily lives. We were constantly on our toes, trying to figure out how to talk with our son and get him to see the big picture. Often, we could not come to an agreement. The phrases, "I don't agree with you" and "We will have to agree to disagree" became useful.

There were even situations when I would look at Justin and say, "I'm going to ignore that statement because it bothers me," and then I'd walk away. This was effective for the talk about being dumb or his expressions of worthlessness.

The walking away part—that was difficult. He would try to suck us right back into the fray of the conversation. Sucking us in reinforced his distorted thoughts, and we could not let that happen. If we reengaged, we furthered his cause and fueled his fire. But it was not easy. I was certain my tongue was going to fall out due to the number of times I was biting it.

Homework was a real problem—a situation where creating a storm could get him out of doing the work. Often, he would complain that it was too hard and say that he was stupid. A typical conversation would go like this:

Seeing Justin going to the fridge for his third snack instead of sitting at the table doing homework, I'd say, "What's going on? You are supposed to be doing your homework."

"It's too hard."

"Can I help?"

In the past, at this point, he would have either manipulated me into doing the homework for him or agreeing to call the teacher because it was too much—which was letting him off the hook.

But a new and improved conversation went like this:

Seeing Justin going to the fridge for his third snack instead of sitting at the table doing homework, I might say, "It is homework time, please put the food away."

"I hate homework. It's too hard, and I'm stupid."

"I'm going to ignore that statement because it bothers me. This is homework time."

I was not supposed to say, "You are not stupid," but I was allowed to say that it bothered me or that I didn't agree. This is a subtle, but important, difference. Telling him he wasn't stupid made him believe I was lying to him. Stating that it bothered me put the onus on me and not him. It gave him no validation or invalidation—but he knew I didn't like it.

The part about not engaging was the most significant. The simple act of engaging essentially gave him permission to fight the battle he was so sure he could win. We could not allow him the platform to dig in and argue his point.

And he would try. He was skilled at twisting everything, so we always had to be on our toes. For example, he would continue the conversation with a statement like, "All I ever do is bother you." This was his attempt to try another path. I learned to respond with statements such as:

"I don't agree."

"I'm seeing you are starting to escalate; do you need to take ten?"

Or I could simply invoke "take ten," but this was also a way to get out of homework, so we had to be careful with this tactic. Instead, I might say, "Justin, I'll talk with you when you are ready to have a respectful conversation."

Another tactic we employed was storytelling—a technique called "Annie Stories." Mary suggested this would be key to getting into Justin's brain. We made up a character named Jerry (nope, not Annie). I would start a story about Jerry, and Justin and I would trade off lines to complete it. It would go like this:

"Jerry had a very bad day at school today. Something very terrible and horrible happened and it was…" And then I'd hand the story off to Justin.

Based on how he would respond, I would add to the story to get him thinking. This gave us the opportunity to present situations from another person's point of view—something Justin rarely thought about.

"Jerry was so mad because Ralph ate all the chocolate cake and didn't leave any for Jerry. Jerry thought about what to do and he…" I'd hand the story off to Justin.

"He told Ralph that it was really mean for him to have eaten all the cake. Ralph said, 'I'm not mean, you are!'" Then he handed the story back to me.

"But then Ralph stopped and said, 'I didn't know you didn't get any cake, so I'm sorry.'" And then it would be up to Justin to figure out how to react.

Sometimes, the stories would be pure fantasy, because we didn't want them to be too therapeutic. If they were, he would stop participating. We would go on "bear hunts" or sail away on a pirate ship to see all kinds of wild and crazy things. When we needed to do something specific, this was a fantastic tool.

Remember the part about my brain being exhausted?

Slowly but surely, we were tackling the mountains. Structure and schedule? *Check.* Calming techniques, language skills? *Check.*

But we still had more mountains to climb.

CHAPTER 16

Making a List

The morning routine in our house was pretty awful. Justin was so slow and unfocused that it started our days on a bad note. To a certain degree, he was manipulating because he didn't want to go to school, and it was his way of exerting his control. It was also a big part of his ADHD.

Mary noted that Justin had a "good competitive" side to him. She wanted us to use it to challenge him to focus. There were two tools we used to accomplish this. The first was consistency, and the second was an egg timer.

Being consistent meant we needed to establish the boundaries and stick to them. We created a rule that Justin was not allowed to be late. The Bachman Bus left for school at 7:45, and if he missed that, he would have to walk. The schedule and lists helped with this.

We continued to include every single step, and we did it with Justin so he could have some ownership. His brain was so disorganized that this was critical. The list started with "Turn off the alarm," and continued with "Get out of bed, go to the bathroom, get dressed, go downstairs for breakfast." It went on to describe every single thing he did in the morning.

This next phase included putting minutes to the list. We did some testing to determine how long each step would take. This gave him a sense of ownership because they were decisions he was making.

This was actually a fun process. We did it on a weekend, and we practiced it so Justin could really understand how long things took. This helped him decide what time to set the alarm. He was able to completely agree with this plan. Not only did he build the plan, but he picked all the goals and the award. This was *his* plan.

We started simple and printed the list with columns so he could check off each thing he did, which gave him a sense of accomplishment.

We started using the timer to help Justin stay on track. In a typical morning, Justin would get up, get dressed, and come down for breakfast. After breakfast, he would go upstairs to brush his teeth and bring down his book bag. This is where the trouble began. Instead of heading into the bathroom to brush his teeth, he would get sidetracked with something.

And this is where the timer came in. Before going upstairs to brush his teeth, I would set the clock for the number of minutes we had noted in the plan. I would say GO and Justin would then race off to brush his teeth. The goal was for him to accomplish the tasks before the dinger went off. This meant he had no time for any distractions.

We started this off with one task at a time. When he would consistently beat the timer with that one task, we would add another. We set milestones, such as beating the timer five days in a row. When he would achieve those goals, he would earn time to play his video games. We never took away video games when he didn't meet the goals. We didn't use any negative consequences because not meeting the goal was negative enough.

When he didn't meet the goal, we let him know to keep trying.

The first few days of the plan went well. We were in the honeymoon phase. Justin owned it and was doing it.

But Justin is a tester, and he knew I would rescue him. After all, that is what I did. My nature is to be a helper. It took me time to realize I wasn't helping him but instead, I was enabling him. When I would let things go, he would seize the day. And why not? Ron was much better at this than I was.

Typically, if Justin ran late, I would pack his book bag or do whatever was needed to get him out the door on schedule. I felt so bad for all the struggles he was facing that I wanted to make things easier. Mary was so nice in explaining how I wasn't really helping.

When Justin slipped back into taking his good old time, I was ready. He missed the timer, and 7:45 came and went. Stef and Konnor had an earlier school start, so they were already out the door. At around 7:50, he came down, ready to go. I followed my instructions to the letter. Here is how it went:

"When are we leaving, Mom?

"Is everything ready?" I said, with my teeth gritted, because I knew darn well it wasn't.

"I don't know."

"Well, check your list."

"Will you pack my lunch?"

"That is your job."

"But I'm going to be late."

"Yes, you are."

He'd start to escalate, saying, "So you want me to go hungry?"

"You being hungry would make me sad. Pack your lunch."

"Fine," he said, as he huffed off to do the task with a loud sigh. "Fine."

After he'd thrown together his lunch, he'd announce, "I'm ready. I'll meet you in the car."

By now it was 8:00, and the first bell is at 8:00, and the second one is at 8:05. "It is after 7:45, so you have to walk."

"But I'll be late." The panic would rise in his voice. "You can't let me be late."

"We all agreed on the rule. If you are not ready by 7:45, you have to walk. You should probably get going if you are worried you will be late."

"I don't know how to get there."

"You can cut through the back yard and use the path through the woods to get to school faster." I slipped here, because he absolutely knew how, but I made a mistake—I wasn't perfect, and I was learning too.

"You can't do this to me! I'm going to be late."

"Then I suggest you start walking."

"Aren't you worried someone will kidnap me?"

"No, I'm not. I'll be right behind you. I won't let you go alone."

"Fine." He stomped off very angry, but there was no storm.

He mumbled under his breath about how mean I was for the entire walk. Of course, he was saying it was my fault he was late. Thankfully, it was only about a ten-minute walk because we lived close to school. I stayed about four paces behind him so I could not feed into his anger, and I was working hard to hold in laughter. The situation was pretty funny. I was so happy that he was handling his anger and that I got him to walk.

About eight months prior, this would have been a one- to two-hour ordeal with a major storm, and I would have ended up driving him to school. We both would have been spent. But not today. After I left him at school, I cracked up laughing as I walked home. I didn't care that I had a stack of work on my desk because now I too was late. I was so proud of both of us. Although I slipped a little bit, I stuck to the plan and so did Justin.

Later that day, when Ron got home, Justin told him the story of what happened, and we processed the things we did well and what could be done differently. There was no outward celebration because we couldn't overdo it, but inside, well, I was doing cartwheels!

We were so sad to see fifth grade end. This team of teachers was so loving and gave so much extra effort to ensure Justin's success. The dream team of Mrs. Miller, Mr. Lyons, and Mrs. Kehoe will never know how truly thankful we were for their patience and understanding.

Justin had gone the entire school year without a single storm. His grades were good.

Hoo-fucking-ray!

Because things had been so hard for so long and we were starting to feel a little bit better, Ron and I decided to take the kids on a vacation. Little did I know I was about to take a leap of faith.

———

CHAPTER 17

The Leap

This was the Bachman Gang's first real vacation—a Caribbean cruise. We signed up for an excursion on the island of Grenada. It was a hike through a plantation—nothing too crazy. I'd made sure it was safe. When we arrived, we started down the trail with a guide and we were able to taste things like cacao and guava straight from the plant. Everyone did it…but me. Too risky. As usual, I was on the sidelines and listened as everyone gushed about how delicious the guava tasted and how the cacao was bitter.

As the hike continued, we arrived at a beautiful waterfall. Our guide indicated the water was deep and if we wanted to, we could jump off the cliff, the twenty-to-thirty-foot high cliff—much higher than the high dive at the pool.

I have *no* idea what possessed me, but I turned to Ron and said, "I'm jumping." He was stunned and looked at me like I had three heads but said, "Okay." I told him the condition was that he do it with me. He agreed.

We made the trek to the top of the cliff. All along, I had carried on a conversation in my head about whether I should turn back. I was so consumed with fear, I was shaking. However, my desire to overcome the fear had grown bigger. I hung back and watched person after person make the leap. Some even came back for a second jump.

I told Ron that he had to go first. I figured that if something happened to him, I could still back out. So, he jumped.

Then, it was all me.

I stood on top of that cliff, looking down at what appeared to be a bottomless chasm.

I was nauseous, sweating, shaking. *What was I doing?* This was crazy. I should back out. But I couldn't let my fear get the best of me.

In that moment, I have no idea what happened or how I made the leap, but—finally—I jumped.

Never in my life have I felt such pure adrenaline. It was a rush. *Wow.* Aside from my marriage vows and giving birth to my three children, this was the greatest feeling in the world.

Not only did I feel adrenaline, I felt accomplishment. I had done it. I conquered a huge fear, and I didn't die! I didn't even get hurt. I did it. I finally left my comfort zone!

That day, I understood that I could do anything I put my mind to doing. I realized how completely irrational the fears were that had been holding me back from so many things, like tasting new foods and meeting new people. Most important, I knew the biggest obstacle I was facing was myself. I was my worst enemy.

Ron and the kids told me they were proud of me for making that leap. Other people on the tour congratulated me because, obviously, they saw what a complete train wreck I was on the way up. But the thing that mattered most to me was how proud I was of myself.

I look back often on the photo of my leap that day. I use it as motivation when my fears rear their ugly heads.

I've learned that the fear will always be there. It comes in the form of hesitation. But I now know it is okay to be fearful. I've learned to use fear more as a barometer to ensure I have appropriately assessed all my risks. I refuse to let it hold me back.

This also gave me the courage to keep going with the hard work we were doing with Justin. We were making tiny leaps every day that were scary as hell, but we would keep jumping. It was working!

CHAPTER 18

The Art of Conversation

Although things were better, the work was not over. Justin still had no friends because his social skills were lacking. Mary had the answer. One of the things she noticed was that Justin was a good talker when it came to things that interested him. However, he rarely took the chance to learn what interested others. He never gave anyone the chance to speak and had a way of ignoring the social cues indicating someone wanted a turn. He was unknowingly blatant about dominating the conversation.

For example, I overheard an exchange between Justin and one of Konnor's friends who was waiting for Konnor to come downstairs.

The friend said to Justin, "Konnor said you watched the basketball game last night; did you see that dunk?"

To which Justin replied, "I got to level five in Mario Kart, and I'm almost at level six."

Often, Justin did not pay attention to what other people said. This was part of his ADHD, but it was also learned behavior that hadn't been corrected.

We got to work.

To start, Mary put some rules of conversation in place. The first was that Justin had to do some research to figure out the interests of another person. We started with easy people—our family. He knew Konnor loved basketball, so his task was to ask Konnor a question about basketball.

Justin was then told he had to really listen to the person's answer, and he had to acknowledge what was being said. He needed to respond with some kind of affirmation and another question.

Konnor was into Duke (which was ironic, because years later, he would become the head manager of the University of Connecticut's Men's basketball team, a rival team). In the beginning, Mary served as a kind of Cyrano de Bergerac and prompted Justin. A conversation would start with Justin asking, "Did Duke play last night?"

Konnor would reply, "Yeah, they won."

"What was the score?"

"Eighty-five to sixty-seven."

"Wow. That's a big win."

And on it went. Justin practiced with our family for several months. Some conversations were forced and seemed like roleplaying, but he needed to do this work. There was something special about seeing these conversations evolve. A few years back, all of his exchanges were arguments, but now, we were talking with each other.

Justin was ready for the next step: the telephone. Mary taught him how to use the phone and how to initiate conversations. His homework was to make one phone call a night. I had to prearrange these calls with people we knew so Justin could practice.

Eventually, the day came when he transitioned to a play date. Ron had reconnected with an old school friend who had recently moved to our town. He had a son Justin's age, and the parents were willing to make a play date. Justin pretended that Mary was his aunt and wanted to take Justin and a friend for ice cream.

Justin had to make the phone call to extend the invitation. Check!

We found out some of this boy's interests and Mary worked to prepare Justin for the big day. Mary picked him up and they headed to Mitchell's for ice cream. We have no idea why, but the first date didn't go as planned. There was a newspaper on the table, and Justin picked it up and read the entire time. Thankfully, the friend had fun anyway, because Mary was there to entertain—but Justin pretty much bombed.

Luckily, these parents were willing to help us keep trying. Mary worked with Justin to process what went wrong. She asked Justin to remember the ice cream date and then they role-played, with Mary pretending to be Justin. She held up the newspaper and ignored him as he started to speak. He quickly got her point; however, getting it wasn't the problem. Doing something about it was going to take a lot of practice.

That's where we were so lucky to have Mary. She wrote scripts with him, and they practiced the art of conversation day after day. Justin was so hyperactive, he was not slowing down enough to listen. Eventually he learned about using deep breathing and focus techniques to stay in the moment and pay attention to the things a person was saying.

Mary and Justin went on more practice dates with friends, then she helped him process how the conversations went.

Developing these social skills was hard for Justin and took years. But it was critical. Not knowing how to interact with his peers led to them making assumptions, and when kids make assumptions, they can be very cruel.

———

CHAPTER 19

Our Gift

Bullying was still a difficult and sad part of Justin's life. It broke our hearts to see such cruelty directed toward our son. We did not witness most of this torment, because bullies tend to inflict harm when they know no one is watching. There are a few occasions that stand out.

Justin played recreational sports, and Ron was always his coach. In the winter of Justin's sixth-grade year, Mary was working hard with Justin on his social skills. We were so relieved—he had come a long way and he continued to be storm free! Although I would not have said he was out of the woods or off suicide watch, we were getting more and more confident that he would get there.

We began to get Justin involved in some outside activities—under a watchful eye, of course. There was a wonderful recreation center in our town with many types of athletic fields, basketball courts, an indoor and outdoor pool, weight rooms, a rock-climbing wall, and it offered activities for people of all ages. This was a place kids hung out.

It was the start of the basketball season, and Ron was coaching Justin's team. Justin had a game one weekend, and I was sitting in the bleachers with the parent of a teammate. Their older son was good friends with Konnor. As the game was underway, two bullies (whom I'll call Dumb and Dumber) showed up to watch the game. They sat right in front of me. Every time Justin took a shot and missed, these children yelled, "You suck, Bachman." At first, I was so surprised these kids were so brazen, I assumed I must have heard wrong.

Nope.

Clearly, they had no idea I was Justin's mom, because they continued their taunts, which shattered my heart each time they called out to my son.

My mind raced. I didn't know what to do. It felt like there was no good solution. I knew Justin heard them, because I saw him glance their way, but he didn't react because he was in play on the court. When he was on the sidelines, the taunting continued. Not once did he look back or react. I was so crazy proud of him for handling this so well.

But how could I let this continue?

I never wanted to yell at a child because I would hate for another parent to discipline my own. I didn't know the parents of these kids, but there certainly wasn't anyone telling them to stop. If I intervened, it might blow back at Justin when I wasn't around. I could see Dumb and Dumber escalating their bullying.

And I had to consider what Justin would want. He was doing so well at ignoring this, and I didn't want to embarrass him. But what kind of example was I setting if I did nothing? The angel and devil were duking it out on my shoulders.

I concluded that if I did nothing, I was allowing this to happen.

So, I leaned forward to tap Dumb on the shoulder, when out of the blue, the parent I was sitting next to looked at me and said, "I got this." It felt as if he had read my mind. He pulled these two kids aside and let them have it. I stood by his side not saying a word but looking like the reinforcements! He then told these kids to leave. Thankfully, they did, but they were snickering and laughing as they walked away.

I felt such gratitude to this parent. For him to stand up for Justin without being asked felt so good. This had never happened before, and I took it as another sign that things were getting better. I figured there could be blowback for Justin, but we could talk about it and plan for how he would handle it.

After returning to my seat in the bleachers, I began to process this situation. These kids were calling Justin "jerky." I had noticed that he was doing something strange with his neck. He was constantly, rapidly turning it to one side. This was something I may have noticed before, but I was really seeing it now.

When we got home, I mentioned it to Ron, and he agreed it seemed odd. We asked Justin about it, and he was unaware. We'd brought it to his attention so he would stop. But he didn't. We asked Justin if something was hurting him or causing him to make this motion, and he said no. We continued to ask him to stop and grew frustrated when he didn't.

This went on for a few days, so we made a doctor's appointment.

Our pediatrician was our first stop. He called it a tic and said it could be a side effect of the Ritalin Justin was taking. But that didn't sit well with us because he had been on Ritalin for three years. Why would a side effect suddenly start? Our pediatrician suggested a neurologist.

Off we went, back to hitting walls in the maze of doctors. The first neurologist told us it was just a tic, probably caused by stress, and that it would pass. She referred us to a psychologist. We were already working with Mary and were thrilled with her, so adding another doc was not going to happen.

We mentioned this to Mary, and she suggested we keep our eye on it for a few weeks, and then we could figure out our next steps.

Engaging our kids in volunteer work was important and Stefanye and Konnor were always doing something. Konnor had engaged with an organization called Friendship Circle where he spent time with a child with Downs Syndrome. As luck would have it, Konnor won an award through this organization, and there was an event coming up, where he and several other kids would be recognized for their service. We received the invitation and saw that it was a dinner, and the agenda included two guest speakers from out of town. I didn't pay any attention to their bios because I knew we were going, and, based on the quality of the organization, I assumed they would be interesting.

Little did we know, this event would be life changing.

As we sat listing to the second speaker, he told his life story about living with a disability called Tourette Syndrome. Justin sat next to me, and I saw that he was completely riveted. Ron and I were as well. So many parts of this speech rang true for us that I was choking back tears. About halfway through the presentation, Justin tugged on my sleeve and whispered to me, "Mom, this is what I have."

The next day, I got on the Internet and researched this thing I knew so little about. I'd heard of Tourette Syndrome because of an old episode of the TV show *LA Law* that featured a character who swore profusely. But Justin wasn't swearing, so I doubted this could be our answer. So much made sense, but so much didn't connect.

We opted to look for a doctor who specialized in Tourette Syndrome and thanks to Google, we were able to get an appointment that week.

The doctor took one look at Justin and knew.

Diagnosis complete.

We could finally put words to what was going on with Justin's body.

And so began our journey into the wacky world of a medical condition called Tourette Syndrome.

The doctor gave us the facts.

Tourette's is a neurobiological condition that causes involuntary movements and vocalizations called tics. Movement tics are called motor tics and can include things like eye blinking, jaw movements, neck turns, arm jerking, hopping, twirling, and many other things.

Vocal tics cause sounds. They can be a sniff, grunt, throat clearing, and can even be more complex and include words and phrases. Because of the way Tourette Syndrome is portrayed in the media, most people characterize Tourette's as the "swearing disorder"—but in fact, only about 10 to 15% of people with Tourette's have swearing tics. This type of vocal tic is called coprolalia.

Tourette's is a spectrum disorder, meaning the severity of the case can vary from person to person. Tourette Syndrome can "wax and wane"—

sometimes tics are crazy big and sometimes, they are milder. Tics regularly change in type, frequency, and severity and can be exacerbated by stress, excitement—you name it, it impacts tics. Tourette's is typically first seen between the ages of five and seven and escalates with the onset of puberty.

This diagnosis was one of those "duh" moments for us. All of a sudden, so many things made sense. The excessive tissue use we equated with allergies? *Sniffing tics.* That neck thing? *A tic.* Justin's case was not in the worst category; however, it was more severe, placing him above the middle of the spectrum. Justin had coprolalia, but it didn't come on right away. It would hit him about a year later, with the arrival of puberty at the start of eighth grade.

We asked the doctor about a prognosis. Would Justin have to deal with this his entire life? He said there is no cure and Justin would live with this forever. However, he told us Justin had a 33% chance his tics would get better, a 33% chance they would stay the same, and a 33% chance they would get worse. We knew nothing.

This was one of those scratch-your-head moments. Should we be celebrating?

The doctor told us that many of his patients have luck with medication, and he wrote us a prescription. He said side effects were rare and that it should bring him relief.

We opted to celebrate and follow the path of optimism—we assumed Justin would be in the 33% that got better. We opted to call this a gift. Yes, it was hard and heartbreaking knowing our son would have to live with this, but after everything we had been through, something finally felt right. We felt like we found the door that led us out of the maze.

We left the office with the prescription in hand, hoping this medication would help and that we were on our way to a better life. This was so exciting for us! We had a diagnosis that made sense and medicine to control it. Justin's therapy was going well, and we looked forward to a return to a normal.

This is where the universe looked down upon us and started laughing hysterically.

Little did we know we had just entered a new maze with a whole new set of challenges to navigate.

Justin started taking the medication and, unfortunately, it did nothing to control the tics. To make matters worse, it had awful side effects. Our highly energetic child was dull and tired. He didn't want to do much of anything. One day, Justin came into my office, lay on the floor, and told me his arms and legs were so heavy that he could not pick them up.

Back to the doctor we went.

He told us that medicating for Tourette's was more of an art than a science. He explained there is no specific treatment and no cure. Many people, especially those with milder symptoms, can use medications meant for things like Parkinson's disease or epilepsy and their tics can be controlled.

We wanted to be positive, so we tried to maintain a good attitude. We went the rounds with four different medications, but nothing seemed to work. Meanwhile, his body was constantly jerking and the sounds were escalating. One day, on a trip to the grocery store, we noticed a man staring at us. We tried to ignore it, until the man turned to us and asked, "Why does your kid feel it's necessary to act like a bird?" and then he turned and walked away in disgust. Justin had this one tic where he would let out a blood-curdling scream—the first time I heard it, I dropped everything and ran, thinking my son was being attacked. No— just a tic. But if he did this in a public space, it was a different story. People would react in all kinds of ways—some nice, some not so nice. I wish I had a penny for every time I got a "stink-eye stare" or had someone tell me to control my kid. If they only knew....

My heart felt so sad, watching a totally different version of our son as he tried to live with the side effects of these medications.

I have always considered myself to be a resourceful person—I am a problem solver—and I realized I needed to do what I do best.

We had not met anyone with Tourette Syndrome, so our pool of people to get advice from was limited. Until this point, we had been private about what was happening behind the closed door of our home. Few people knew of Justin's suicide attempts or the therapy we were going through.

But this was different.

We knew Justin would have to live with this his entire life. Even more, the tics were so obvious, they couldn't be hidden.

We remembered that we found Mary through a friend in the special-needs baseball league. This would be a safe place to start. After all, they were a group of people who may not all have experience with the same condition, but all understood life in the maze.

When we mentioned Justin's diagnosis at one of the games, a mom told us about a friend of hers who lived in another state. Her daughter had Tourette's, and she was willing to reach out to this mom to see if she would talk with me. When I heard that, I was so excited I couldn't dial the phone fast enough! I was so eager to learn and had a million questions.

I wanted to understand how she explained this to other people and how she acclimated her daughter in school. Were they experiencing the same issues with medications? What types of advocating did she do and how did she build her daughter's confidence?

When she answered the phone, I introduced myself and told her I was so excited to talk with her and—

She cut me off.

I didn't get to ask her a single question.

She took over the conversation and was adamant that we tell no one. She said we should pretend Justin didn't have Tourette's and that we should hide it from the school because he would be labeled. She told us it would be a preexisting condition in his medical records and cause us problems.

She didn't have a single positive or helpful thing to say.

After I hung up the phone, I was a wreck. This was the worst advice ever! How could we hide this? Our son was a walking bundle of erratic movements who blurted out body parts and swear words. There was no way we could hide this. And we didn't want to.

I thought hard about the idea of Justin being labeled. Ron and I talked about this for a long time, and we spent a good amount of time processing it with Mary. One of the first things she suggested was that we really think about the word: *label*. She asked us if we considered a person who was deaf to be "labeled." In this context, it was obvious—of course not. Tourette Syndrome was a diagnosis, not a label. Labeling was something other people would do—something we would have no control over.

As we continued on our journey, the concept of labeling came up many times and it was something I began to feel strongly about. I believe labeling is a dangerous thing people do when they make invalid assumptions.

Fuck labels.

So, we kept going. We started asking more and more questions and doing more research.

I found a book that had a character with Tourette Syndrome—*A Test of Will* by Diane Shader Smith. The author's website listed her address, so I sent her a note asking if she would talk with me. To my great joy and surprise, she wrote me back with her phone number and told me to call her anytime.

We had the most wonderful conversation! She gave me hope. She suggested I call Judit Unger, Executive Director of the National Tourette Syndrome Association in New York. Judit was her friend, and she said I could say she referred us.

At first, I was reluctant to call. I assumed this would put me in touch with a support group. I am not the "support group" type. I felt guilty that I felt this way, but I knew this wasn't for me. Don't get me wrong, I know a lot of people truly benefit from these groups, but I just couldn't make the connection for our family.

After a lengthy conversation with myself, I figured I'd call anyhow. We had already been down so many paths leading to nowhere, what was one more? The worst that could happen was that I'd turn back around in the maze. I reminded myself that this was for our son, our beautiful boy who deserved something good. We were always encouraging him to keep a positive attitude, so how could I make assumptions and not even investigate a new possibility because I thought it might be another dead end? I told myself not to give up on the hope that maybe, just maybe, this could be different.

Boy, am I thankful I gave it one more try. This turned out to be our best game changer yet!

I dialed the number expecting a receptionist to answer and give me the third degree—this woman was a high-level executive of a national organization. I assumed she had much bigger fish to fry than to talk with me. If the receptionist didn't give me the third degree, then the executive assistant surely would. But I was prepared. I had the name of her friend, and I was going to play it close to the vest. I was simply going to say, "Diane suggested I call" and leave it at that.

As expected, a receptionist did answer. I asked to speak with the Judit Unger, and I heard simply, "One moment please." I listened to the hold music as I waited for the assistant to give me the runaround, but much to my great surprise, Judit answered the phone.

But wait… I hadn't planned for this!

I went silent and didn't know what to say.

In fact, she had to repeat "Hello" three times before I gathered my wits about me.

Looking back, I really should have known better than to make assumptions. Lesson learned.

I started the conversation by telling her about Justin. I'm not sure what made me do this, but I started pouring out my heart. I cried and talked and sobbed and talked and then cried some more.

The amazing thing is this: she listened! She took time from her busy day to listen to every single word I said.

I told her about Justin's suicide attempts and how I felt like the worst mother in the world. I told her how lost we were and that the medications were not working. I told her we felt so alone because we didn't know anyone with this condition—and how we had been fighting, but we were so tired.

She kept listening.

She didn't interrupt me.

Not once.

She just let me spill my guts over the phone line.

Of course, she was acknowledging me. She was empathizing every step of the way, and she made me realize there was help available to our family.

Somehow, she knew when it was appropriate for her to talk. She told me she was happy I had called and that she would help. We had been on the phone for more than an hour, and we continued talking for about another hour.

Suddenly, I realized I needed to take notes. This woman was a Godsend and in my deeply emotional state, I realized I needed to write things down. I did not want to forget a single thing she said!

I took about ten pages of notes during our conversation. She told me about so many things. She suggested books to read and movies to watch. She sent me a whole packet filled with information about how to explain Tourette's to the people in Justin's school. More important, she told me that the association had certified people in every state who would be willing to come into Justin's school to help the team understand Justin's condition. And there was no charge for this! Wow! Free help to have someone come to the school—how could this be?

She told me there was an Ohio Chapter, but it was based out of Cincinnati, which was about four hours from us. She gave me the name of the chapter leader and suggested I call her, because they did have activities throughout the state.

The best thing she described was their National Youth Ambassador Program. Without having met Justin, she suggested he apply and said he had a good chance of being accepted. The program admitted new "classes" every year. State chapters invited people to apply, and every state accepted one or two students between the ages of ten and eighteen. The state had the funds to fly each student and one parent to attend a four-day program in Washington, DC, where the students and their parents would learn about advocacy. Then, everyone spent a day on Capitol Hill. This sounded right up Justin's ally!

Actually, I take that back. The best thing she told me was that she would be there for us, and that any member of our family could call her or anyone on her team whenever we needed something. And, let me tell you, through the years, she made good on that commitment! She returned every single call we ever made. *Every single one.* Like Mary Poppins before her, this woman was an angel who changed our lives.

Judit sent us a card. She explained that people with TS often endure strange stares and intrusive questions. The National Tourette Syndrome Association had cards printed that we could hand out.

WHY DO I ACT THIS WAY?

Because I can't control it

I have Tourette Syndrome, a medical condition. It causes me to make loud sounds, have twitches, and say things I don't mean. I can't help it any more than you can stop a sneeze. I'm sorry if it bothers you—it bothers me more.

This busy woman put her entire day aside not only to talk with me, but to listen. I made a vow to myself that I would be just like her. If anyone was ever in a situation like mine, I would be their person. And I have made good on that promise.

____

CHAPTER 20

Back to Earth (With Some Tools This Time)

After getting off the phone, I called Ron to tell him about the amazing call I had. He was so happy to hear me sound so excited. I'd been excited before, only to have my hopes dashed, but this was different. I could feel it in my bones. This was real.

We were looking forward to Mary's next visit. I could not wait to tell her about all these resources. We'd finally found a way through the maze!

True to form, Mary brought us back down to earth and had us take a step back—or, as I like to say, we had to "restrain our enthusiasm."

Mary reminded us that one of the ways we had pulled Justin out of his dark place was by letting him own his problems. Because Justin had to live with this diagnosis his entire life, he needed to have control to navigate how he did things.

She was so right. I couldn't start handing out these cards without his permission. The last thing I needed to do was embarrass him! And while the Youth Ambassador Program sounded great, he needed to *want* to apply.

So, we brought Justin into the conversation, and I explained all I had learned about the National Tourette Syndrome Association.

Thanks to our education from the doctor, Justin was aware of his diagnosis. I explained that we needed to figure out how to live with it—all five of us—but he needed to take the lead. We told him that it was his job to figure out how he would manage. It would be his responsibility to tell us how to help him as well. We outlined that we were still the parents in charge, so sometimes we would give him choices, and there would be instances where we would have veto power. But for the most part, he was in the driver's seat.

This was right around the time Justin started a new medication. The side effects were the worst yet. Not only did they make him tired, but he was constantly nauseous and throwing up a lot. Talk about pathetic and heartbreaking.

The timing was quite opportune! As we were discussing his newfound power to own decisions about living with Tourette Syndrome, he ran to the bathroom to lose his lunch yet again. When he came back, he announced that this would be his first order of business—no more medications.

He was done, over it.

He told us: "I feel like a science experiment gone wrong. The meds are not making the tics go away, so there is no reason for them."

We told him we agreed with his decision, but that we needed to talk with the doctor to ensure we stopped the medication the right way. I didn't want him to go cold turkey if that meant something bad could happen. I scheduled an appointment, and soon Justin began living without any medication to control tics. He stayed on the Ritalin to help his ADHD, but otherwise, he was med free.

Justin was receptive to our plan. He was thankful we were putting him in charge. We explained that he had grown and matured. Most important, we were beginning our third year of being storm free, of being suicide-attempt free.

We used the word "suicide" with him. We told him how proud we were that he chose to work hard to get better rather than ending his life.

We did explain that with each decision, there would be natural consequences—some we might be able to plan for and others we might not be able to anticipate. But we knew that if we worked together, the Bachman Gang could deal with anything.

Justin decided he wanted to use the cards from the National Tourette Syndrome Association, but he didn't want to be the one to hand them out. Ron and I agreed to carry a stash with us, and we would use them when we deemed it appropriate.

We reflected on the many times people had given us strange looks or said something about the way Justin was acting. Justin said that if the cards would stop people from saying those things, then he wanted us to hand them out. He said maybe that man from the grocery store a while back would not have been so mean if he understood Justin's condition.

He was right! These cards were wonderful. They gave us freedom. We had not been to many restaurants because we were afraid of the stares. Now we had a tool. When we handed the card out to tables around us and let people know they might hear and see some strange things, people got it. For years, we used these cards in all sorts of places and people thanked us and told us they understood.

___

CHAPTER 21

Finding a Role Model

Justin was about to enter the eighth grade, and we learned that the elementary school psychologist had moved up to the middle school. This was concerning because we'd had nothing but problems with that team. We decided to call the school to ask for a meeting.

We had some decisions to make. We really didn't like the way our son was treated back then. Would this woman be able to undo the label she stuck on Justin? We also did some soul-searching and realized it was a two-way street. We had come far as a family, and had to take some responsibility of our own.

During the meeting with the assistant principal, we expressed our concerns and also our understanding. We talked about all the success Justin was having, and he encouraged us to engage the school psychologist in an open and honest conversation. She would be an integral part of the team, so it was important to make things right with her.

So, we did. We called the meeting and had a productive conversation. We embraced the idea that some of our issues were of our own doing. We asked her to forgive us, and we forgave her. She never came out and said she had labeled us as bad parents or Justin as a bad kid. I have no idea, but I'm guessing she made assumptions about us that were not favorable—we had certainly made those assumptions about her. We'd assumed she didn't care. Just as she was wrong, we were wrong too.

After that meeting, she would turn out to be one of Justin's biggest advocates.

Justin was on an IEP, and the school psychologist was going to lead the charge to make the updates to accommodate his diagnosis of Tourette Syndrome. It is classified as a disability, and he was eligible to receive services.

One of the suggestions I got from the National Tourette Syndrome Association was to watch a movie called *Front of the Class*. This is the true story of a man named Brad Cohen, a person with Tourette Syndrome. It was the story about how he became the teacher he wished he had. We asked Justin's teachers to watch this movie. Some did and some didn't, but it was all okay.

True to my nature, after watching the movie, I wanted Justin to meet Brad! So, we got online and Googled him, and sure enough, we found his foundation. Brad's email was on his website, and we sent him a note. To our shock and amazement, Brad responded within minutes and was willing to speak with us!

I was again so impressed by the sense of fraternity from these people we were meeting. First, author Diane Shader Smith, then Judit Unger of the National Tourette Syndrome Association, and now Brad. We were finally feeling blessed.

We talked with Brad for a bit, and he asked Justin some questions. He learned that Justin liked to play the clarinet and he was just starting to play the saxophone. Brad asked Justin to write up a profile and to send Brad a picture so he could share it on his website. How cool—this famous person wanted to put Justin on his website. Amazing!

Brad also told us about a camp he founded called Twitch and Shout. It was a weeklong camp for kids with TS that took place during the summer. Hundreds of kids would come from all across the country. I could not sign Justin up fast enough! It was only September, but Justin looked forward to that day in July when he would board a plane to Atlanta.

CHAPTER 22

Bar Mitzvah with Tics

In the Jewish faith, when children turn thirteen, they enter into adulthood in the eyes of the religion by participating in a Bar (for boys) or Bat (for girls) Mitzvah. The children study with their rabbis and learn how to lead a Jewish service, culminating in reading from the sacred Torah scrolls, an incredibly high honor.

Family and friends attend the service, which is typically followed by a huge celebration. Justin was working hard to prepare for his Bar Mitzvah. We were lucky to have highly caring Rabbi Rosie and Cantor Kathy to help. We joined the temple when Stefanye was in kindergarten and I was pregnant with Justin, so both Rabbi Rosie and Cantor Kathy knew us well. As it turned out, Ron and Kathy were old high school friends. We had a great team!

Justin would turn thirteen in June, but for a variety of reasons, we opted to wait until September of his eighth-grade year to hold his service. This would give him extra time to study.

When Stefanye and Konnor were in seventh grade, they both received many invitations to Bar and Bat Mitzvahs. It seemed as if they were going to one or two services and parties almost every week.

This was not the case with Justin. One of our neighbors had a daughter Justin's age, so we were all invited to her Bat Mitzvah, but that had been his only invitation. Until one day an invitation arrived that was solely for Justin. You can't imagine how excited he was to get this in the mail! It was for a Bat Mitzvah for a girl he really liked. He ripped open the envelope, asked if he could go, and of course, we said yes! He had me fill out the response card to be sure they could read his name, and he ran at top speed to get this back in the mailbox so they would know he was coming.

Justin marked the date on his schedule, and for about a month, he counted down the days.

His joy was so real, and we were thrilled for him. Things really were turning around.

Until they weren't.

The roller coaster turned us upside down.

About two weeks before the big event, the phone rang. It was the mom of the girl having the Bat Mitzvah. She was calling to tell me that Justin should not attend because of his Tourette Syndrome.

I immediately assumed she was talking about the service and that Justin's tics could throw off her daughter's concentration during an important moment. I explained that I would attend the service with him and we would sit in the back row. I assured her we would leave if his tics became a problem.

That's when she said, "No, you don't understand. He should not come at all."

I was speechless. I honestly didn't know what to say. So, I just said, "Okay."

I remember sitting on the bed staring at the wall. I have no idea how long I sat there trying to process this—but it was a while, because Ron came looking for me.

I asked him to close the bedroom door so we could talk privately, and I told him what had happened. He was as stunned as I was. Neither of us had any idea how to handle this.

No matter what we did, our son would be devastated.

Now I was angry. Did she have any clue what she had just done? If they didn't want him to come, then why invite him in the first place?

Who does this?

How could an adult be so horribly cruel to a child?

I wanted to attribute it to her ignorance, but I couldn't. If it were simple ignorance, she would have asked questions and shared concerns—but no, she didn't want to hear my explanation or come up with a solution. This was blatant disregard of our son's differences.

I had to process my anger. In the privacy of my home, I could call this bitch every name in the world, and I could have pure hate for her. And boy, did I ever! This was that awful Mama Bear anger I had not felt in years. This was "protect my son from the pure malice of the world" anger.

After yelling at Ron and getting it all out, I was able to calm down. I needed to move on from the rage and figure out a plan. I could see Justin's happy face the day the invitation came, and I visualized him running to that mailbox with so much excitement.

Shit.

There was no right way to handle this. It was a complete no-win situation.

We brainstormed all kinds of solutions. We could call the mom back and try to reason with her. But why would we want to put our son into a situation where he was not welcome? This woman was ballsy enough to call us, who knows how she or the other kids would treat our son. This was not an option.

Neither Ron nor I had the heart to tell him about the phone call. How do you sit your child down and explain that he is unwanted? We had just gotten him to the place where he had moved from feeling unwanted to feeling loved. We could not put him back there.

Ron and I decided we needed a break and tabled the decision. The event was two weeks away, so we had some time.

As luck would have it, the next day, Justin got into a little bit of trouble. We had told him he was not allowed to have a Facebook account, but a little birdie told us he had created one without us knowing. This was a huge *aha* moment for Ron and me. We decided that the consequences of breaking our rule would be that he would not be able to attend the Bat Mitzvah.

Of course, he was angry, but he had broken a rule and knew there would be consequences. He handled it as well as could be expected, which of course made it even harder for us.

We opted to still send the girl a gift. After all, we had no idea if she knew what her mother had done. We took the high road and mailed a card with a check. We knew it was received because the check was cashed. Sadly, we never received a thank you note, but we didn't do it for that reason. I still feel it was the right thing to do.

Although we tried to protect Justin from knowing about the phone call, he was smart enough to figure out that we had used the consequences from his mistake to protect him. Years later he told us he knew something was up and we told him about the phone call. The remarkable thing was, he appreciated what we did—he was really growing!

As a result, we lifted the penalty and told him he could do whatever he wanted that night. Times like this really confirmed how the years of therapy made a difference for all of us.

Justin really did like this girl, and when he was making the invitation list for his Bar Mitzvah, he wanted to invite her. He was a much bigger person than me! We said it was perfectly fine and sent her an invite. She RSVPed that she would come, and Justin was really excited. We did tell him not to be surprised if she didn't show, which is exactly what happened.

Our journey with Tourette Syndrome impacted every aspect of our lives. Preparing for Justin's Bar Mitzvah was no different. During the service, Justin would be required to hold the Torah scroll and read from it. It is the holy scripture to be held with the highest respect. Thankfully, we were close with our Rabbi and Cantor, Rabbi Rosie and Cantor Kathy.

We treated his Bar Mitzvah training just as we did school and requested a meeting to educate them about Justin's tics.

I don't know if it was hormones, or nerves about the upcoming big day, but Justin started to tic the word "bitch." When he would practice for his Bar Mitzvah, he used this word while holding the Torah, which is completely unacceptable. Because we took the step of education, Rabbi Rosie and Cantor Kathy understood these were different circumstances and they let him hold the Torah and read from it. A huge honor!

Justin had taken up the saxophone and whenever he played the instrument, his tics would stop. We thought that if we incorporated the instrument into the service, it might help calm the tics. Justin and Rabbi Rosie worked together and selected a prayer, and Cantor Kathy got him the sheet music. Although he still "tic'ed" throughout the service, this gave him a tiny bit of respite and it added a truly beautiful moment to his service.

We made an entire weekend out of this celebration, and it was fantastic. It was also my parents' wedding anniversary, so we were able to celebrate with our out-of-town family as well. It was such a great time for Justin to be in the spotlight.

Amidst all the preparation and activity, we paused to reflect and realize what a pure miracle we were living. Justin was alive and had triumphed over so many struggles and was approaching not only this day, but a future no one anticipated. This religious moment let us count the blessings of our children and Mary and how we had scaled a huge mountain.

We had so much more to celebrate as our son met this milestone of entering adulthood in the Jewish religion. He did a beautiful job, and the party was plain fun. We purposely tried to do things differently from other parties to add some novelty with a "Jamaican Me Happy" theme and a DJ we brought in from out of town. We didn't invite hundreds of kids, but the kids who came really made Justin feel special.

It was magic.

All around it was perfect.

But you know what happens when things are perfect.

The wind blows in a new direction, and the roller coaster takes a new turn.

In our case, it meant it was time for us to say goodbye to Mary. She needed to open her umbrella and fly on to a new family.

We were fearful of losing our safety net, but we always knew Mary was only a phone call away. Our last session with her was emotional. She gave us the "you've got this" speech and we reminisced about her first day with us sitting on the floor outside of Justin's bedroom. We didn't know how to say goodbye, so we didn't. I held her tight, reluctant to let go, without saying anything. We cried together, she pulled away, turned around and walked out the door. This isn't supposed to happen with a therapist, but we felt a strong emotional attachment to her. She had spent so many days at our house, staying hours. She felt like a member of the family, and we kept in touch for a while, but in the end, she let us grow on our own. Mary gave us a gift we will never ever forget. She taught us the tools we needed to get our child back.

Would we be able to stand on our own for what was to happen next?

CHAPTER 23

Life After Mary Poppins

The vibe in our home was new. Although focused on the impact and intricacies of Tourette Syndrome, we were able to enjoy the excitement ahead for our older kids. Stefanye was in her junior year of college, and this turned out to be the year she met the man of her dreams, Matt. Konnor was beginning his senior year in high school and had applied and been accepted to the University of Connecticut and Indiana University, and we were eagerly awaiting his big decision. Konnor had moved on to a new group of some really terrific friends. It was sad that the friendships he had with the Magnificent Seven completely fizzled. I had hoped that, as things got better for us, those friendships would return, but they didn't.

That was fine. It had to be fine.

Thankfully, Konnor was so social and friendly that he moved on. High school was a great experience for him. Almost every weekend, our home was filled with his buddies who chose our house as their hangout place. It was a beautiful noise I would miss when the kids went off to college.

What was amazing was that they were all so accepting and kind to Justin. They looked out for him and treated him well. Ron and I tried hard not to let Justin infringe on Konnor's time with his buddies, but it was nice to know that once in a while, they didn't mind.

Although we were still vigilant, the fear of suicide was no longer at the forefront of our lives. We were still dealing with a lot, but Justin was safe from self-harm.

However, he was still highly disorganized. Losing things was a constant, and he hated to read and write—school was not something he enjoyed.

We were still adjusting to Tourette Syndrome, but Justin had a great toolkit and felt more confident than ever about advocating for himself. He decided he would take ownership of the cards, which was a giant milestone. We could sense his pride whenever he handed one out.

As puberty set in, Justin's tics got worse. They were much more physical, and boy were they loud! At this point, he wasn't swearing or blurting out words, but we lived with a lot of screeches and some strange noises.

Watching our child's body contort in ways we knew it shouldn't was terribly difficult. These tics were becoming much more prominent and a huge source of worry for us. It is heartbreaking to know your child is in constant pain.

Oddly enough, Justin didn't complain. This made it even harder for me! You have to love the resiliency of a kid. It's not that I wanted him to complain, but I realized that I was struggling with this so much, it would have made things easier for me if he were complaining. So, on top of the worry, I felt guilt.

I was happy not to fear for my child's life, but now I hated the fact that he was hurting.

Never a dull moment.

Never.

I had to constantly remind myself that this was not about me. Yes, it was hard for me, but I had to follow Justin's lead. I had to understand that if he accepted this and was rolling with it, then I needed to do the same.

If it didn't bother him, why should it bother me?

I struggled. My only answer—because I was his mom. What parent wants to see their child in pain? Ron struggled as well, but he seemed able to deal with it just a bit better. That was good, because I could rely on him for strength.

One day, I was reading comments on Facebook, and I saw a post written by a mother who has a child with Tourette's—a few years young-er than Justin, really a great kid who was smart and bright, one you fig-ured would do really great things.

She started her post with a "long rant." She went on and on about how difficult things were for her. When I first started reading, I empa-thized and totally got it. She was talking about my life!

She went on to vent about how much she hated Tourette Syndrome. *Preach, sister!* I'm with you!

But then her post took a turn. She said her child had accepted their tics and was fine with them, but she wasn't. She described how much she hated her life, asking why she was chosen to have to deal with this child. She questioned how her child would ever make it in life and had resolved that she was in for a life sentence with this child living in her house forever.

Her post read, "Who would hire such a weirdo?"

I was taken aback. As parents, we have to understand that our kids pick up on so much from us. How can our children believe in themselves if we don't? How can you encourage your child to apply for a job when you believe they won't get it?

My heart broke for this poor woman, but it broke into extra pieces for her child. I totally understood where she was coming from—to a point. This is hard stuff, and she had every right to feel angry, sad, and any other emotion she was experiencing.

But…

I hated the fact that this woman posted negative things about her child on social media. I'd seen it before and still see it frequently. I see parents calling their children lazy or discussing things that simply should not be discussed in a public forum.

No parent should ever post anything angry or negative about their spouse or children on social media.

Never.

Never ever.

All I could think about was what would happen to this child if they read the things their mother had posted about them? In this case, it was a private group, but her child was a member!

I've seen similar comments posted publicly—some about TS, some about other things. I've seen posts from moms publicly berating their children for not calling home.

Let's turn the tables. What would happen if our children posted about their parents' awful behavior?

In that moment, I realized this woman had not moved into the acceptance phase of dealing with the giant monster called TS. I couldn't judge her because I know how tough this all is; however, it made me realize that if I didn't accept every single thing about my son, he would feel it.

I began to understand that my fears for Justin were being projected outward and subconsciously affecting the way I acted with him.

I remembered being a first-time mom and having someone tell me that if I was anxious when I held my baby, the baby would feel it. This was no different. I considered the times my kids fell and skinned their knees. They would look to me to see how they should react! If I returned an "Oh no!" expression, they would cry, but if I said, "You're good" and helped them get up, they would brush it off, say "I'm fine, Mom," and keep going.

If I was projecting worry about Justin's pain or negativity toward TS, he would feel it.

If I wanted Justin to be successful, I had to believe he would be successful with every ounce of my being.

I also had to stop taking on pain on his behalf.

When he told me, "I'm fine, Mom," I needed to believe him.

CHAPTER 24

The Catalytic Moment

Thanks to my conversation with Judit at the National Tourette Syndrome Institute, we were much better prepared to start the eighth-grade school year.

During our meeting with the school psychologist and assistant principal, we asked that a meeting with Justin's teachers take place before school started. We had never done this before, and for the school, it was an unusual request. Justin's teachers told us later they had never been in a meeting like this. Thankfully, the assistant principal was happy to comply because he knew the teachers had never taught a student like Justin.

The school psychologist, Justin's interventionist, and the guidance counselor attended as well. We were thrilled to have the guidance counselor there because he was also the cross-country coach, and Justin would be on the team again. He had run in seventh grade and enjoyed the sport and the comradery he shared with his teammates.

In the spirit of continuing to allow Justin to own his destiny, we asked him how he wanted to handle the meeting. He decided that he would hand out the cards with information about Tourette Syndrome to the teachers, but he wanted Ron and me to run the meeting.

When we walked into the room, the teachers took one look at Justin and were stunned. His tics were so severe that they blatantly stared at him, unsure of what to do. You could feel their uncertainty.

We kicked off by providing an overview of Tourette Syndrome in general, and then we got specific about how it impacted Justin. We gave them insight into how the tics felt and the way they could be especially distracting in terms of learning. We asked them to ponder this: "Imagine you are reading and approximately every twenty seconds, someone lifts your head away. Then, you have to find where you left off each time." We painted a picture of exactly how Justin processed, or didn't process, information.

We told the teachers that blurting out the word "penis" or dropping an f-bomb might seem funny, but to consider what it was like when it happened all the time. We didn't want pity, but we needed their empathy to motivate them to ensure Justin's success in the classroom.

Some of the teachers later told us they thought they knew what Tourette's was, but they admitted this was different. They all appreciated our information.

Then, something great happened—the teachers started asking questions.

"Do you know when the tics are happening?"

"How can we help you without embarrassing you?"

The teachers were on our side! Hello, collaboration!

Seeing the willingness from the teachers gave Justin the confidence to speak up and participate—to advocate for his own needs.

As part of Justin's IEP, he was allowed to leave the classroom whenever he felt he needed a break. He was entitled to teacher notes and lesson plans. The teachers suggested it would be best for him to be at the back of the room; however, Justin explained this would be harder for him. He spoke up and told them he was concerned the other students would constantly turn around every time he tic'ed. Justin also noted that if he was close to the door he could easily slip out with minimal interruption. Everyone agreed.

We were aware that Justin's tics were highly unusual and shocking to people who were unfamiliar with them. Although he never intended to interrupt, we knew sudden loud noises could bring any room to a halt.

We recognized this would be hard for the teachers to deal with and we wanted them to know this wasn't a one-way street. Justin would need to make accommodations to help them as well.

To deal with this, we came up with hand signals the teachers could use if Justin didn't realize he was tic'ing repeatedly. To keep embarrassment to a minimum, the teachers would simply walk by Justin's desk and tap on it. This was a signal for him to get up and stretch or to tic in the hallway. If Justin missed the signal, the teacher would suggest he get a drink of water.

We added a line to Justin's IEP that required he take tests in a private room so he did not disturb other students. Removing Justin from the classroom at times like this was the best option.

After discussing teacher accommodations, we talked about the most important thing: the students. We knew if we educated the other kids, they could understand and help by not making fun of something Justin could not control. So we provided each teacher with this script:

Many of you know Justin Bachman, but some of you don't. From time to time, you will hear him make some strange sounds, say inappropriate words, or you may see him make some spastic-looking movements with his body. Justin has a medical condition called Tourette Syndrome. The movements and sounds he makes are called tics.

There are a few things you need to know:

- *He cannot control these sounds or movements any more than you can stop an itch or a sneeze.*

- *Sometimes he can hold them in for a little bit, but if he does, they build up and come out later much worse.*

- *They are not contagious; you can't catch them.*

- *He is still the same typical kid, just like all of you. He is in the marching band and is an important member of our class.*

What each of you can do:

- *Don't be afraid to ask questions.*

- *Treat him like you always have.*

- *Try and ignore the tics if you can.*

- *Remember that he wants to stop the tics way more than you want him to stop.*

We asked each teacher to read this script on the first day of school, and we asked them to do this before anything else. We wanted the teachers to read it because they were in a position of authority, and we knew the students would listen. We also requested that the teachers provide students with five minutes to ask Justin questions. He was happy to be completely open and would answer every one.

At the conclusion of the meeting, Justin spoke and told the teacher his goal was to make his tics like the air-conditioning noise. He explained that you hear the air conditioner turn on, but after a while, you get used to it and you don't pay attention.

We left the meeting with a spring in our step. It had gone exactly as we had hoped.

The first day of school rolled around, and I was a nervous wreck for the entire day. Were the teachers reading the script? Were the students being cooperative and listening? Would any of them make fun of Justin? I think I felt every tick of the clock go by. I couldn't wait to jump into the car to go pick him up.

When I saw him walk out of the school building, he was smiling!

I immediately asked, "So…how'd it go?"

Thankfully, he was his usual chatty self and gave me every detail. He told me all the teachers complied with the plan and read the script.

That is, all but one: the cross-country coach.

The script had worked. The kids asked some good questions, and there was not a single one that stumped him. He was surprised when one kid asked if Justin would die from Tourette's, but he realized it was a valid question. He was happy to answer with a firm no!

Justin mentioned that the cross-country coach didn't say anything to the team, and I asked him how he wanted to deal with that. Justin said he would remind him the next day, but he figured most of the kids had heard it already, so he was covered.

Eighth grade cross-country meets took place on weekdays right after school; however, we were told that there was a large invitational meet coming up in mid-September, on a Saturday. This was a big event that would include thirty teams from all over Northeast Ohio.

Unfortunately, it fell on the Jewish holiday of Yom Kippur, which happens to be the holiest day of the year. We were torn about what to do. Justin really wanted to run and be with his teammates. Attending temple services was difficult for Justin because it was hard for him to be quiet, and the Yom Kippur service is somber.

As a family, we emphasized that the holiday was important. We went to temple for the Kol Nidre services on the Friday evening before Yom Kippur, and we decided Justin and I would go to the meet on Saturday while Ron and Konnor would stay home and go to temple. Stefanye was away at college.

Justin was so thankful we were letting him skip temple to run. He boarded the team bus with great enthusiasm.

I found my way to the finish line so I could be there to cheer for Justin. While we were working on getting Justin well, we had withdrawn from the social scene, so I wasn't "friends" with anyone on the team at that point, but I knew who they were and had nice acquaintances with several of the other parents. I stood next to a couple of them, and we chatted as we waited for the boys to come in.

I had no idea what was happening at the starting line.

Gene was the first of the kids to cross the finish line, soon to be followed by Alan. Both the boys were breathing so hard and looked like they had run the race of their lives. When their parents saw them coming, they were thrilled and noted that they were finishing faster than normal.

Gene came over and grabbed my arm. Alan went to his mom. I could see on both their faces that something was terribly wrong. But they were so tired from running that neither was making any sense and could barely talk. All I heard was "Justin."

My heart stopped. I assumed he had fallen, so I asked, "Is he hurt?" Gene shook his head, and I could hear Alan's mom telling Alan to calm down. Gene started to drag me over to the track as he pointed at something—I had no idea at what, but he was clearly pointing.

All of this happened in a matter of seconds, but to me, it felt like hours. I was in a total panic, and it took every ounce of energy to be patient and let the boys tell me what happened.

Finally, they told me Justin had been disqualified because of his tics.

My first reaction was relief. I asked again if he was hurt, and they said no. They were not sure where he went, but they were going to go back to find him.

This is what I loved most about the team. The kids were so supportive of each other.

Justin knew I'd be waiting at the finish line, so I figured between him knowing where I was and the boys looking for him, he would eventually find me.

My next thought was that kids are dramatic, and it couldn't be that bad. I was just happy he wasn't hurt, so I began to calm down.

Gene showed me who the officials were, so I figured I'd go talk with them to get their side of the story while I waited for Justin. There were two of them.

I walked over to where the men stood and calmly introduced myself. I said, "Some of the boys on my son's team told me there was a problem with Justin and that he was dis—"

I never got to finish my sentence.

One of the officials looked at me and said, "Oh, there was a problem alright."

Now, I knew my son. I knew the tools we'd equipped him with to deal with situations where he had to advocate for himself. I responded evenly and explained, "Justin has a medical condition, he—"

I was interrupted again.

I will never forget what happened next. I can still close my eyes and see these men. One of the officials looked directly at me and said, "Lady, I'm a special education teacher, and if your son was retarded, I would know. Your kid is rude."

I was stunned for so many reasons. First, no one calls me "lady." Who the fuck did this guy think he was?

And worse…the R-word. What kind of "educator" would ever use that term?

For the first time in my life, I had a great retort. I looked him square in the eyes and said, "I'm thrilled you are not my son's teacher." I went on to tell him—not ask, but tell him—I was going to find my son and then they were going to apologize.

Without waiting for a response, I turned and walked away in search of Justin.

I'm not sure what came over me, but I remained calm. I walked a few steps and saw the boys with Justin. He was sobbing. I mean ugly-cry sobbing—shaking, red-faced, and snot everywhere. I held him for a minute, and we didn't say anything. I just let him get his feelings out.

When he was ready, I pulled out of our hug and dried his tears. I said nothing and waited for him to speak. He didn't say much but he told me he was embarrassed and upset—he was afraid the team would lose because of him.

I told him I had spoken to the officials, and they were going to apologize. I took his hand and we walked over to where these "educators" stood.

At this point, Justin's teammates and their parents had gathered around and were watching us. They moved in our direction but kept their distance. It was an eloquent show of support.

I introduced Justin by name to these men and told them he was ready to accept their apology. They told us they had nothing to apologize for. I was stunned, but I knew I needed to be calm for my son.

I asked them for their names, and they refused. Justin looked up at me and then at them. As they started to walk away, Justin said something so profound…it's something I'll never forget.

As I'm sure you have gleaned by now, our son is never quiet. It's not in his DNA. He is loud and boisterous, but not this time.

I heard a little voice.

It was almost like Cindy-Lou Who from *How the Grinch Stole Christmas*, but the volume increased as he spoke to these officials, saying "If you won't give us your names, you must know you are wrong."

They turned to look at him. They heard, but they continued walking away.

As the officials skulked off, all of Justin's teammates gathered around and asked if he was okay. The parents from our team were furious. They'd heard the exchange and were in the same state of disbelief I was. I had parents of boys from other teams approach me to tell me their sons had told them what happened and how wrong the officials were.

One mom and her son came over. When she found out they hadn't given me their names, she asked if I'd taken a picture.

Why hadn't I thought of that?

I could worry about it later. I had to focus on Justin. He wasn't talking at all, and I could see his tears had returned. They were no longer sobs, but tears continued to fall. He looked like a zombie. I had a horrible dread he was returning to the dark place.

I knew I should have asked him if he wanted to ride on the bus with the kids, but I could not let him go. I needed to be with him. I told him I wanted him to ride home with me.

He didn't argue.

He didn't say anything, just continued to grip my hand.

Justin's coach was not there that day, and the coach of the girls' team was responsible for all the kids. We walked over, and I signed a form saying I was taking him and that he would not be riding the bus.

We said our goodbyes to the other parents, and we left.

It was about a forty-five-minute ride. Justin and I drove in near silence the entire way. I asked a few questions, but he didn't answer.

I was angry, but this was not the time. I needed to give him space to feel his emotions.

When we arrived at home, Justin went straight to his room and closed the door. I told Ron about what happened, and we cried together. I told him I was so afraid and that we needed to check on Justin. We wanted to give him his space, but we needed to be sure he was safe.

We had our extended family coming over for the traditional Yom Kippur dinner to break the fast. Should we cancel? There was no good answer.

Ron and I asked Justin to come downstairs so we could have a conversation. We sat at the kitchen table.

At first, we all looked at each other with expressions of helplessness. Things had been going great—his classmates were understanding, he was finally doing well in school. Justin had built up a foundation of confidence after the diagnosis—yet in an instant, it felt like the walls had crumbled around us all.

But we had to move forward. Mary was still with us in spirit, so we pulled out every tool from her toolbox!

Ron and I started the conversation by explaining that what happened to Justin was wrong.

So wrong.

We explained that anyone who can't admit a mistake is weak.

But we had no control over those officials, so we needed to focus on how we were going to deal with this situation.

We told Justin that he was entitled to feel every single emotion he was feeling.

Ron and I explained that there are people in this world who simply won't understand his condition. Sadly, something like this was bound to happen again. Because of this, he was going to need a plan for how to cope in the future. We brought up suicide and reminded Justin this was not an acceptable solution. We told him we would give him time to process everything and in the spirit of letting him control the situation, we asked him how many days he needed.

Justin was not being conversational at all, but he listened to everything we said. He told us he needed three days. We have no clue how he came up with this number, but he did, and we went with it.

But there was a deal to be made. At the end of the three days, we would all gather back at the kitchen table, and he would need to tell us his plan for moving forward.

That night, our family came over, but Justin stayed in his room. We checked in on him periodically, but we gave him his space. Of course, he had to go to school, but at home we didn't bother him.

This was tough. I wanted so desperately to ask how he was feeling, but I didn't. I wanted to hug him, but I could only do so if he asked for one, which he did on a few occasions. We really and truly left him alone.

On the third day, something happened that had never occurred before.

CHAPTER 25

Lemons and Lemonade

The phone rang. It was for Justin!

Some of his teammates called to see how he was doing. I wanted to force him to come to the phone, but we couldn't do that. I was so excited kids were calling, but this wasn't about me. We promised to let him deal with this in his way, so we had to make good and keep our word.

If he was up for talking on the phone, he did, and when he wasn't, we thanked the kids and let them know we would give Justin the message.

The phone rang for us too.

This simple act of people calling to check on us meant the world. This was a horrible situation, but good was coming from it.

Many of the people who called were encouraging us to file a lawsuit claiming discrimination. Although we appreciated their recommendation, this was not something we were interested in doing. Emotionally, we could not handle a fight.

But we knew we needed to take some kind of action. During our three-day "sentence of silence" with Justin, I called the school to discuss the situation with the athletic director. I told him we wanted to get in touch with the right people to request that officials (*all* officials, we were not singling out the two offenders) be trained on compassion and how to handle students with disabilities. Based on the behavior of these two officials, we figured there had to be other kids out there who, for whatever reason, had faced intolerance.

More important, we said we would bring in a trainer at our own cost. We didn't want them to be able to use the excuse of expense not to do it.

Sadly, the athletic director was not much help. He told us he was sorry about what had happened, but there was not much they could do. He told us we could call the Ohio High School Athletic Association and suggest it to them.

That is exactly what we did!

I tried to speak with the top person, but I could not get past the gatekeeper. I was instructed to file a formal complaint.

So, we did.

Once we filed the complaint, I received a call from an employee of the Athletic Association, asking for my side of the story. They claimed they knew nothing of the incident but would investigate. I reiterated our desire to provide free training. I said I was not looking for anything other than the opportunity to ensure this did not happen to another child.

A few days later, we received an official letter in the mail from the Ohio High School Athletic Association stating there was no proof to substantiate that the incident occurred.

This was another stunning moment in our lives. How could they deny that it even took place? We had so many witnesses.

We felt we were being very reasonable. We didn't sue, all we wanted was education. But these assholes decided to deny the entire situation ever happened.

Disbelief.

This was a blow to the gut.

Thank goodness we had gone through all the therapy, because it made it easier for us to realize that we could not control their actions. Not easy, but we were able to work through it.

We had to give up on them, but by no means were we giving up!

On Monday, when Justin came home from school, I wanted to ask him about what the kids had said, but I needed to give him space, so I didn't. It really was killing me not to bombard him with millions of questions. But I zipped it shut.

When he woke up Wednesday morning, Justin told Ron and me he was ready to have a meeting with us after school.

This was so cool! The process was working. We made good on our commitment and now, Justin was making good on his.

Later that day, Justin sat Ron and I down at our kitchen table.

He began to explain that the thing he remembered most about what happened was that his teammates stood up for him. Even though their advocating didn't work, they still did it. He realized they were able to do that because we had educated them.

He went on to tell us that all the education we were doing ahead of time was working. He noted that the coach was the only one not to read the script, and more important, he noted that the coach should have educated the officials ahead of time. We could not guarantee this would have avoided the problem, but we felt pretty confident that we would have had a different outcome if the officials had been educated prior to the race.

He told us he was still angry with the officials, but he realized that in their defense, they were uneducated. As Justin put it, "Education overcomes ignorance."

He then laid out his plan.

First, he wanted to be sure to thank his teammates for the way they stood up for him. He would later use the term "Up Standers." We decided I would call our local newspaper to see if they would do a story on the situation and also call the school principal to see what she would do to acknowledge the students. I felt this was a wonderful teaching opportunity to recognize a group of kids who had done the right thing. Sadly, the school principal refused to hear anything and did not want any part in thanking the kids.

We thought we were on our own.

Again.

That's when I heard from the newspaper. They were excited to tell this story! I called the school to let them know a reporter would be coming to practice and was told that the school wanted no part in it.

I would not be deterred!

I called all the parents individually and asked them if their kids would be willing to stay after practice to talk with the reporter. Every single one was thrilled to participate. The reporter took a picture of all the boys, and we were able to get the kids the recognition they deserved.

When the paper came out, we were so happy to see the picture was printed on the front page! This was so cool. I got extra copies and personally brought them to the next meet, and Justin handed them out to the boys with yet another personal thank you.

The next part of Justin's plan was even more spectacular.

He told us he wanted to hold an event that would educate people, and he wanted to call it the Tolerance Fair. He used the word "tolerance" because it is a starting place on the road to respect and acceptance. Anyone can be tolerant. (Remember, he was only in eighth grade when he came up with this!)

Justin had done some research, and he presented us with a list of fifteen charities that included organizations like the Tourette Syndrome Association. He wanted each of these nonprofits to set up a table and invite people to meet their organization so they could inform participants about three specific topics:

1. Educate: each organization would educate about the population it served. In other words, Autism Speaks would educate about autism, and the UpSide of Downs would educate about Down Syndrome.

2. Resources: each organization would promote the types of resources available to people impacted by each condition. Justin knew how much the Tourette Syndrome Association helped

us, so he wanted to be sure people in other situations would know how to find help.

3. Volunteer: each organization would showcase opportunities for people to get involved. For years, our family had been volunteering with a number of organizations, and we learned so much from that involvement. Justin wanted others to be able to know what was available to them.

Ron and I were so proud of him. Of course, we told him. We asked him how he was going to go about holding this event. And he said he wanted to call the Mayor of our hometown of Solon, Susan Drucker. We had not met her, but this was the first step.

In keeping with our commitment to let Justin own his plan, we let *him* call Mayor Drucker to schedule a meeting. Her scheduler was excited that a thirteen-year-old kid was interested in meeting with the mayor, so she got us on her calendar that same week.

We all went to the meeting, but Ron and I simply provided transportation. Justin took command and told Mayor Drucker his story. She was touched and said she absolutely loved the idea. She offered to let us use the Solon Recreation Center as the venue at no cost.

This was a victory! The event was on.

We picked a date and Justin got to work.

This was right up my alley as an event planner, but I had to let Justin do the heavy lifting. This was his solution, and he would need to be the one to implement it. So, we sat down at the kitchen table again, and we asked him a lot of questions.

In the back of my mind, I knew he had a list of fifteen organizations. I figured that maybe half would return his call and he would be able to get his teammates and our neighbors, family, and friends to come. My expectation was that if we had thirty people, it would be a great success.

We asked him how he was going to get the organizations to register, and he responded he would call them. We discussed what the room would look like, and he said he figured each organization would need a table. Great.

We talked about how he would get people to participate. He said he would make a flyer, invite his friends, and ask them to invite their friends.

What happened next was a series of events we never would have expected.

We had a tiny setback in January. Justin was sledding with his friend, and somehow, the sled slipped and hit Justin below the knee. This resulted in a fracture of the growth plate on the tibia. The challenge was that Justin's tics were so severe, he could not be casted. The doctor designed a brace that would give the leg enough room to tic but still keep it immobilized so it could heal. He gave Justin a cane to use, which Justin affectionately named "Herman."

Crisis averted.

Justin got on the phone and started calling the organizations. Many were so surprised to hear from a thirteen-year-old kid, they took his call.

He was also persuasive. There was no cost to the organizations to participate, and the event could only have an upside.

Justin had an idea about how to entice the organizations to participate and ensure they didn't decline his offer. He asked each one to put together a prize basket worth $100. They didn't have to buy anything, but he encouraged them to put something together that would draw people to their table. Each exhibitor would have a box for raffle tickets. When people entered the event, they'd receive a bag to hold all the literature, a booklet describing each organization, and an explanation of the raffle.

Justin knew that people wouldn't be interested in visiting the tables that didn't apply to them personally, but he wanted them to learn about each organization. He figured the raffle baskets would encourage everyone to at least stop by each table to get educated.

Justin made calls after school, and when he left for school the next morning, he would remind me that if anyone called back during the day, I should tell them he would call them back after 3:30, when he got home. He decided he would do his homework after dinner so he would be able to make his calls while people were still in their offices.

The remarkable thing was that everyone called back. Not only did they call back, but they suggested more organizations for Justin to call. And they asked for flyers so they could help with promotion.

We were starting to see that this little event he cooked up was taking off!

Suddenly, the press was calling. Every single TV station in Cleveland wanted to interview Justin, which was publicity we so appreciated.

Because it was getting so big, we knew we needed help.

Stefanye was away at school, so she was doing her best to help from afar. Both she and Konnor tapped into their friend networks to help us get volunteers. They were both so amazing in wanting to support their brother.

Konnor was part of the high school newspaper, and his advisor let him write a couple articles. He wrote about the travesty of the cross-country meet, and he planned to publish another piece after the fair. We always knew our kids were protective of each other, but it was so beautiful to see Konnor's passion to help his pain-in-the-ass little brother. You just didn't mess with Justin in Konnor's eyes.

We figured that if we had half a dozen organizations, we could print the programs ourselves at home. But with the number growing every day, this task was getting too big for Justin to handle. We sat down and had another discussion about how we could get some help. We asked my employees and some friends to be on a committee, and they were all happy to join in.

One of my employees designed the program booklet and got information on printing. Others helped us get food donated, so now the event included free food!

It started to feel as if things were playing out like the movie *It's a Wonderful Life*. We had been through so much, and to see people and organizations wanting to work with us was surreal.

Now, instead of Justin reaching out to organizations, they started calling us. One woman who called to tell us about her organization and ask if she could participate said they had goggles people could wear that would simulate the feeling of a brain injury. There was an organization that made adaptive wheelchairs that asked if they could facilitate wheelchair basketball games in the gym.

This was unbelievable!

The day before the event, Justin was still getting calls from organizations who wanted to have a table. At this point, I was helping with the calls because it was just too much for one child to handle!

We didn't have any kind of an RSVP system, so we had no idea how many people would come. I increased my prediction from thirty to around a hundred people, but Ron and Justin knew it would be a lot more. I was still apprehensive, but who was I to burst his bubble?

The day of the event, we had forty-eight organizations registered to exhibit and sure enough, someone showed up at the door asking for a table.

Not only did the rec center donate the venue, but they donated tables and chairs and offered to help us set up. We arrived early to ensure we were ready for the arrival of the organizations and the food.

When I tell you we used every inch of that rec center, I'm not kidding!

To our surprise, people who wanted to attend were lined up outside the door an hour before the start of the event! There were so many people, the exhibitors who arrived during the later part of the set-up time had difficulty getting through the waiting crowd.

Before the event even started, there were more than a hundred people waiting.

Holy cow!

When we opened the doors, the people started pouring in. It was just incredible.

Cleveland is a town divided into east and west sides. Rarely does anyone cross over, but they came for our event. We met so many west siders who wanted to see what this was all about.

The atmosphere was electric. I cannot even begin to describe it. People were happy and excited. They were learning. They were meeting each other and making connections!

This was unbelievable.

Every local media outlet, the TV stations, our main newspaper, and several other local publications sent reporters to cover the story.

They saw people navigating a wheelchair obstacle course to better understand what it feels like to live life from a wheelchair. There was the brain injury simulator. A group of special-needs people performed a play about bullying, and a beautiful group of women with Down Syndrome, called the Singing Fingers, performed songs in sign language.

People came up to us and thanked us for putting on this event. We heard so many stories. Some were sad, but they were grateful to have come to find help. Others inspired us with their strength and compassion.

People also wanted to give money. We had to make an immediate decision about what to do, because we were not a nonprofit and could not legally accept donations. We ended up dividing the funds among all the nonprofit exhibitors—each one received a check!

Every single table had activity. Many of the organizations told us this was one of the best events they had ever attended and that they'd collected more names than they had at any other. This included the two suicide prevention booths. And as we suspected, they were among the busiest tables.

People were registering for services and making volunteer commitments. Organizations developed partnerships. The Girls Scouts struck a deal with an organization called Hattie Larlham so they could do regular volunteer work.

Individuals became inspired to take on special projects. We met a teenager who ended up designing and building wheelchair-friendly picnic tables for one of the organizations.

And there were more projects and connections made that we would come to hear about through the years.

The rec center staff told us that more than a thousand people had attended. At one point, the Fire Marshall wouldn't let people in because we had exceeded the occupancy limit. I have never been happier to eat my words. Ron and Justin were right—we certainly had more attendees than my anticipated one hundred.

The success of the event made our hearts sing. It was unbelievable that an idea formed at our kitchen table and thought out by a thirteen-year-old kid could accomplish so much.

In the days immediately following the fair, we felt like celebrities. Everywhere we went, people approached us to either thank us or tell a story about someone they met or something that came out of the fair. We heard from people who tried to attend but could not find parking.

I still don't have the words to appropriately describe the magic that happened that night.

The most important result of the fair was the surge in Justin's confidence. This was a high you couldn't get from any kind of drug. Little did we know things were about to get even better!

————

CHAPTER 26

Youth Ambassador

Earlier in his eighth-grade year, Justin was accepted into the National Tourette Syndrome Association's Youth Ambassador Program, and the week after the fair, we would travel to Washington DC.

This was another life-changing moment. Little did we know that this program, combined with the cross-country meet and Tolerance Fair, would completely change the course of our lives.

The association paid for Justin and one adult, so we opted to drive to Washington, DC and paid the fee for meals so both Ron and I could all attend.

Before the trip, we had to participate in a few conference calls. During the calls, we learned we would be taking a day to go to Capitol Hill to meet our senators and representatives. The woman who ran this part of the program was a dynamo! Elridge was amazing. She provided us with letters to mail and let us know she would be scheduling meetings for us. She explained everything we should expect to happen. We were so excited and did exactly as she instructed. It were as if she lived in our house and knew Justin needed a detailed schedule.

The anticipation for this conference was sky high. The excitement brought so much happiness into our home. We were finally going to meet other families just like ours.

When we arrived and checked in, we were greeted by Tracy and Val, who were energetic and encouraging. They gave us packets, explained the entire schedule, and let us know where we needed to be and when.

Then, we got to meet the Executive Director, Judit. Although we had only talked on the phone up until this point, I felt like she was my best friend. I hugged her with every ounce of love I had to give. She spoke with Justin, and they bonded. Years later, when Judit retired, Justin would be one of a few kids asked to speak at her party. She truly meant the world to us.

The conference had barely started, but we felt like we were home.

We were immediately surrounded by people who understood. For the first time, Justin met other kids with Tourette's, and we met parents. We arrived on a Tuesday evening, and the first event was a mixer. They had the kids go into a different room, and they did icebreakers.

They had accepted forty-five kids into this program. I don't remember how many states were represented, but I believe it was around fifteen. There was one other student from Cincinnati representing Ohio, and we were excited to meet the family. Most states had one student, but states like California, Texas, and New York had three or four.

I typically am not thrilled entering a room filled with total strangers, but this was different. Everyone was so eager to connect. I ended up meeting four women, all from different states: Autumn, Cindy, Tammy, and Patti. They became my new sisters. We don't see each other often, but we still communicate regularly and are lifelong friends.

There were some dads there, but few. We are always surprised at how many moms end up dealing with these issues on their own. We heard stories of dads who simply didn't want to admit their child had anything wrong or were not involved. Although I've always been thankful for Ron, this trip made me realize even more how lucky I am to have a life partner who is present every single day.

At the end of the evening, we met up with Justin. "Wound up" was an understatement. I had no idea how he was going to sleep. Needless to say, there was no problem when the alarm went off the next morning— Justin sprang out of bed, ready to go.

The morning programs started out with information about Tourette's. Although we knew a lot, there was so much more to learn. Although the courses provided great information, meeting similar people provided the lessons. We knew that tics were different for every person but witnessing it in the kids made it real. One child had a jumping tic. Every few minutes he would jump out of his chair. Another child was constantly banging his head on the table. Some were hitting themselves and some would go up to people to randomly poke them. There were many different words being blurted out at any given moment.

At first, my heart was breaking. I felt so much of the pain I knew these children dealt with every single day of their lives. It was physical and mental, mostly because of their tics, but also because of the stares, jeers, and bullying that came from the uneducated people outside our safe little circle.

But quickly, I learned not to feel sorry for them. Ron and I saw resilience like never before. No matter what, they were still kids. Real kids with strength and determination to live a normal life. They were the ones who totally owned this disorder and were not about to let anything get in their way.

After the first hour of the training, Judit, the Executive Director, addressed the attendees. Her speech was a statement we will never forget. She stood up and told us her goal was for every kid to leave knowing their tics were irrelevant. That was one of the most powerful things we heard.

She gave every person in that room the ability to live like any other person. She absolutely acknowledged that TS is considered a disability, but it didn't mean life was limited. She specifically mentioned that Tourette Syndrome posed no limitations for success. She went on to talk about people with TS who were doing spectacular things, and she noted we would get to meet some of those people throughout the conference. There were athletes, chefs, actors, entertainers, businesspeople—there was nothing, absolutely nothing, that should limit anyone's aspirations.

The entire room was so energized and motivated—I swear, if I had to run a marathon, I could have done it.

I looked over at Justin and saw a child with a completely new lease on life. The relief and joy on his face made Ron's and my hearts soar. I cannot even begin to describe how empowered we felt. We all needed this. We deserved this.

The afternoon session was dedicated to the kids learning a speech they could use to advocate for themselves and educate others. This part of the program was taught by students, so the kids in attendance really got it. They spoke the same language. The kids broke up into small groups to learn how to give this presentation. It was unbelievable. The kids caught on and learned so quickly. I realized that because they lived it, the memorization was easy.

Meanwhile, the adults were all getting to know each other. Throughout the years when Justin was on suicide watch, we felt so isolated and so alone. Ron and I learned that many of the kids in the room followed similar paths. Not all of them had contemplated or tried suicide, but they suffered and felt lost, outcast.

If only we had known each other sooner, maybe we could have lessened some of the pain. But you can't go back, and we knew we had to move forward.

My new sisters and I began to formulate an idea. We never wanted anyone to have to travel the path we had walked alone—all of us experienced the same struggle to find resources. This was around the time Facebook was becoming popular. Tammy was more educated about its use and suggested we form a group called "Tic Talk." She took it upon herself to create the private group and asked us all to contribute. It was a beautiful new way to find, receive, and offer support. Today the group has thousands of members. To Tammy's credit, she still puts her heart into the group and helps people every single day. She is my hero.

At the dinner on Wednesday night, we were given instructions for the next day: Thursday was advocacy day. This was something special!

We were a bit nervous, but Elridge took all the nerves out of everything. Her planning was so detailed. She left nothing to chance. We were given maps, a schedule of appointments, and scripts for what to say. We were told to give our Senators and Representatives what was called a "Dear Colleague" letter—a letter explained that we were advocating for funding for Tourette Syndrome research from the CDC. Their signature on the letter would provide their support.

Justin stayed up a little bit to hang out with his friends, but we called it a night early to get ready for the big day.

Teal is designated the color of Tourette Syndrome, so all the boys were given teal ties and the girls, teal scarves. Almost 200 of us got on buses at the hotel and exited at Capitol Hill. We ended up being slightly delayed because we had to pause and wait for a motorcade to pass transporting the Queen of England!

When we arrived at Capitol Hill, we took a group photo on the steps of one of the capitol buildings. Then we went into a briefing room where several senators and congresspeople planned to have lunch with us. Justin was selected as one of three students to go up to the podium and tell their story. This was a huge honor.

He got up to speak and stood at the podium with the government insignia, looking like a dignitary. He was composed and spoke beautifully, with a confidence we had never seen before. My eyes could not hold back the tears of pure joy. We had no clue at the time, but this was really the beginning of Justin's career path.

After lunch, we all went in our own directions to our meetings. Because we were advocating at the state level, we spent the day with the other family from Ohio. They were wonderful. Their son was a bit older than Justin, and his case was much more severe. It was one of those situations where you wanted to succumb to heartbreak, but their strength simply would not allow it. At the time we met them, they were searching for answers. In the upcoming years, this child and his family would endure at least three deep brain simulation surgeries, with minimal relief.

But this never stopped him. His ease came when he played piano. And, wow, could he play! He went to college, and he did well!

Our first stop on the hill was to meet Congressman Steven LaTourette. Of course, his name was funny, and the first thing Justin asked was, "Do you know you have Tourette in your name?" He answered that yes, he had heard that a few times!

Congressman LaTourette was amazing. He sat and intently listened to the boys tell their stories. There were questions, and he told us he would absolutely support our Dear Colleague letter.

This felt like such a victory! We'd had no idea what to expect. Before this, we had never met one on one with any elected official, and we had no idea if he would challenge us, disagree, or give us lip service, but he was so genuine.

Oh, wait—there is more!

As we were wrapping up, Congressman LaTourette asked us if we would like a personal tour of the capitol. We immediately accepted. One of the office workers made himself available and guided us all around the capitol building. He took us into rooms that were not on public tours, gave us all the history, and told the stories of things that happened in each room. Most important, he really rolled with the boys' tics. We noticed he was simply ignoring them and treating them like any other person. It was the perfect experience and added another great memory to our trip.

Thankfully, our meetings were pretty spread out, so we had the time to take this tour, but it meant we had to hustle to get to the meeting with our senator.

Sadly, this meeting did not go as well. I'm not going to name the person in office at the time because I don't want this to seem political. Unfortunately, when we arrived, we were told that the senator would not have time to meet us, so we were going to sit with one of his aides. They showed us to a meeting room and, although we were right on time, they left us waiting for over half an hour.

This woman walked in, sat down, looked at her watch, and said, "You have ten minutes." She didn't say hello or introduce herself, but she made us aware that we were a major inconvenience to her day.

The boys launched into their speech, but it was obvious she was not listening. She continued to check her watch and at about the nine-minute mark, she announced that the senator did not commit to Dear Colleague letters. She thanked us for coming and she left.

We were all pretty frustrated and sat there for a moment in disbelief. At least this meeting was the second and not the first. The aide had been so rude and uncaring. Chalk it up to a life lesson. We told the boys to focus on the great meeting we had with Congressman LaTourette and that not every meeting was going to go their way. We noted we were so proud of how professionally they behaved. Although the woman wasn't listening, they had a job to do and would not be deterred by her rude behavior, and that was to be commended.

Everyone gathered at the hotel, and we all shared stories of our day on Capitol Hill. We went to dinner with our new friends and continued to enjoy every minute.

We now had a new family, our Tourette Syndrome family. These were friends we would rely on, who truly understood and could empathize with every facet of our lives. I could pick up the phone and call any of my newfound sisters to express frustration or seek support, and they would really get it.

Because there were so few fathers, Ron didn't have the same experience, but he still felt the sense of family with all the girls and the kids. Ron is a big kid, so he bonded with every single one of them, but I wished more dads had participated to set a good example for their children.

We have great friends who don't share our TS experience, but there is something that goes above and beyond when you share a common but unusual part of your lives. It's an understanding on a different level and something you should seek out if you don't have it.

Many of the national associations for all kinds of conditions (like autism and epilepsy) hold conferences and have special programs for kids.

We highly recommend seeking out these organizations. They may not be as life changing as the National Tourette Syndrome Association was for us, but they have access to many resources. Whether local or national, these conferences provide the opportunity to meet people wearing shoes similar to the ones you walk in every day. Meeting people who truly get it is worth everything. We stretched to afford some of the conferences, but it was worth every single penny.

But the best was for Justin. He loved this trip more than I can describe. When a child suffers from something like TS, meeting people who are just like you is invaluable. These kids bonded so quickly. Nothing mattered—they all liked and enjoyed each other in a totally judgment-free space. We were incredibly proud of the big shift in Justin's mindset. He was no longer the victim who hated himself, but was growing into an enthusiastic leader who would know how to handle the many ups and downs on his continuing rollercoaster ride.

It was so special.

This made it hard to leave. Justin cried and felt disappointment in his heart that it would be a while before he shared the same space with his friends.

Ron and I held him and encouraged him to have his feelings. There was no denying this was sad, and he was allowed to feel sad. We gave him the space he needed, and we talked about how we would move forward. We were thankful for texting and social media, which would be the next best thing.

We all promised to continue going to the conferences year after year, and we did!

After being so sad to leave the conference, Justin knew he had more excitement on the horizon. Thankfully, several of the kids he met in DC would be going to camp, and it made him happy to know he would see them in the summer.

CHAPTER 27

The Challenges of a Disability

Eighth grade was a pivotal year for Justin. After our meeting with his teachers before school started, they all looked out for him and were highly dedicated to ensuring his academic success. The hardest subject for Justin turned out to be language arts. Between the attention issues of ADHD and the disturbances of the tics, reading and writing were difficult. Justin had little to no interest, and his grades reflected this.

Enter Mr. Paris! He figured out how to reach Justin by focusing on things that interested him. The class was working on poetry and Mr. Paris spent a lot of time with Justin, asking questions to help him dig deep within himself to express his feelings. Justin wrote a poem that surprised us all!

Living life different

Living with tourette syndrome is like going through life
with a permanent kick me sign on my back.

There are days standing in the cold i just want to go mad.

I feel like this will be forever.

Like i will never change.

But me making noise, konnor studying hard,
mom working full time.

These will always be.

I am thinking there is no turn at the end of the road,
a dead end, all i can do is disappear.

But if i try to disappear i will always be heard.

It was a beautiful new beginning. Mr. Paris researched books that had characters with Tourette Syndrome and purchased them specifically so Justin would have something pertinent to read. Justin moved from low grades to earning As and developing a love for writing. Mr. Paris will never know the depth of our gratitude. He is the teacher who changed everything and set the stage for Justin's career as a brilliant writer and storyteller.

Although Justin's social skills were still lacking, he had two buddies from the football team. While we were planning the Tolerance Fair, the school was planning the eighth-grade trip to Washington DC. Justin was excited about the trip, and he made plans with one of these friends and another student to be roommates. I completed all the necessary paper-work. Because we were friends with the parents, I had some conversa-tions about them being excited to room together.

Shortly after the fair, I received a call from the teacher who was in charge of the trip—a teacher I knew well. Justin was in his class, and he had taught both our older kids. I cannot imagine how difficult this call had to be for him since he was a huge advocate for Justin.

He was calling to tell me that the paperwork turned in by Justin's buddies specified other students as roommates.

Nobody requested to room with Justin.

That smacked us back to reality.

I did what I always do and figured there must be a reason. Perhaps they were afraid Justin would tic in his sleep and keep them awake.

Because one of the moms was a good friend, I decided to call her to see if I could understand their concerns. After all, this was pretty new to all of us and hard to understand. With all the new tools I had learned, I knew I could approach the situation from a much more collaborative head space. I opted to work it into one of our conversations.

She brought up the DC trip and asked me if I was going to the informational meeting. I said I was, then mentioned, "I know we said our boys would be rooming together, but it seems that is not the case." I left it at that, and she immediately said she thought they were rooming together as well. She said maybe the school changed things around and that she would check with her son to be sure he was rooming with the kids of his choice.

I was so relieved. I had a good conversation where I was able to share concerns in a productive way. I was learning! I was confident this would get fixed.

But it didn't.

She never called me back.

At first, I told myself to give her some space. This issue was far more important to me than it was to her. Although, I did feel that her son's treatment of my son was significant, I told myself to be patient. I also didn't want to be annoying and was trying not to be angry.

I wondered if she was embarrassed and perhaps we didn't need to have another conversation because she would simply take care of it.

About three days later, I was notified by the teacher that we had to figure out the roommate situation. There was one room with an open spot, and he had called the parents and thankfully, they were willing to have Justin room with their boys.

I felt smacked in the face once again.

Ron and I talked about it, and we opted to just let it go. There would be absolutely no benefit in forcing anyone to room with Justin. The consequences of that could be much worse.

But we were so disappointed in our friends.

If the mom had called me back and just said something—anything—I would have had more respect for her. To simply ignore the situation and our feelings felt like a punch in the gut. We deserved more respect.

We sat down with Justin and talked with him about it. We told him that people don't always make sense, and we were going to have to be okay with that. We didn't have to like it or agree with it, but we could not let it set us back. We decided that instead of focusing on the unanswered questions, we would move on and figure out this roommate situation.

I hated feeling like a charity case. To have to ask someone to be with our son was so painful, but Justin rolled with it and wanted to go on the trip. Justin knew the boys he'd be rooming with—not well, but he was fine with it. They were nice families, and we worked hard to focus on the good stuff. At least he would be able to go on the trip and have student roommates. We framed this as an opportunity to make new friends.

Phew!

Problem solved.

Sort of.

Justin was hurt. This was the beginning of the end of the friendship with the old buddies. Our saving grace in this situation was that it was more about young teens trying to figure out where they fit in. It wasn't about our child acting poorly. This is something that was bound to happen at some point, Tourette Syndrome or not, and it is the type of hurt every kid faces. As we were accustomed to doing, we picked ourselves up and started moving forward down a new path in the maze.

Thank goodness Justin had the tools for this. Difficulty happens to everyone. Friends come and go, but when you have a child who has attempted suicide and has mental, medical, and physical issues to deal with—well, that's a whole different ballgame.

I didn't see it then, but now I realize this was the first time we had to deal with a typical kid problem. I wish I'd been able to give myself that perspective at the time.

Whenever something like this happened, I would hold my breath and pray for Justin's strength. Ron and I could not solve his problems, but we could ask him to tell us how he was doing and how he was handling things. If Justin opted to provide detail, which he often did, our job was to listen. And if he didn't provide details but told us he was handling it, we had to be completely fine with this. If he told us he had it, we had to believe he had it.

We had a bit more preparing we needed to do for Justin's school trip to DC. Because of the experience at the cross-country meet, we knew prior notification about TS was important. The teachers in Justin's school were so wonderful and helpful. They provided me with the itinerary, and we worked together to figure out what parts of the trip could be difficult.

The one that stood out was the visit to the US Holocaust Memorial Museum. This was a quiet, somber place where Justin's TS could cause problems. I called the museum and spoke with their guest services team. I gave them all the details about Justin's upcoming visit, and they were wonderful. They indicated they would notify their security team and we should be fine.

And he was—in terms of security, but not in terms of his psyche.

The museum visit took a toll on Justin. The Holocaust Museum is difficult for anyone, Jewish or not. Being Jewish, this had a bigger impact on Justin. It is the story of our history; one he had been taught at a young age. Ron's father had been on the Kindertransport, and Justin knew the stories of many Holocaust Survivors.

As they entered the dimly lit room, all the students were quiet. The tour guide began talking and used the word "Jew," which immediately signaled Justin's brain to tic that word. His loud tics echoed through the quiet room. He stood frozen, hating Tourette Syndrome.

As the tour continued, words like "kike" and "Nazi" spilled out of his mouth.

In Justin's mind, tic'ing through this museum felt like an uncontrollable attack on his own people. The emotion of it all was overwhelming, causing him to cry, which further aggravated his tics—the perfect storm.

When we first got the diagnosis of Tourette Syndrome, we were so relieved to know what was happening to Justin that the reality of living with it didn't sink in right away. His first tics were more motor oriented, and the first vocal tics were sounds, but now he was tic'ing words and phrases, and this felt different. People assume you can control words and sounds that come out of your mouth. People can understand uncontrollable movements, but language paints a different story.

Having words come out of his mouth that he would never speak voluntarily brought a new set of questions. How could his body utter such words in such a sacred place?

And there was absolutely nothing he could do about it.

Nothing.

This event brought all of us to somewhat of an emotional standstill.

How do you handle it when something inside your brain forces you to do something you feel is unforgivable? There is no medical or logical explanation why people with Tourette's tic the words that come out.

There was nothing we could do but keep moving forward with the knowledge that, if given a choice, these were things Justin would never say.

We were beginning to understand the enormous importance of the power of advocacy.

We had always advocated for Justin, and it took on many forms—whether it was for services he needed at school or medical advice. But this was different.

Because we had prepared the museum's security team, he was not punished or victimized. His teachers and trip chaperones were also supportive. The seeds of education we planted were growing and fostering Justin's personal safety and acceptance. I always worried, and still do worry, that someday he will unintentionally utter something offensive, someone won't understand, and the consequences will be bad.

There was something else that happened during the museum tour that caused us to pause.

We used a lot of coping mechanisms to deal with Justin's tics, and humor was one. Many of Justin's tics are funny—he can tic the word "bitch" at just the right moment to be funny—and we wanted people to feel comfortable laughing with us. Ron is fantastic at using humor, and so we rolled with it—we laughed. The tics could be funny!

But this was different. Some of the kids on the trip thought Justin's tics at the museum were something to laugh at.

And so, they laughed. It wasn't intentional, but it was not appropriate.

How do you mitigate that? How do you determine when it is okay to laugh and when it isn't? The answer to this question should be clear cut, but it is not.

This hit me hard for a number of different reasons. When we received Justin's diagnosis, we felt it was a gift—and for many reasons, it was. It allowed us to understand things about our son.

We all accepted this as a lifelong diagnosis, but this was the first time I saw Justin feel so bad about tic'ing. I imagined myself standing in a courtroom and a judge banging down a giant gavel as he imposed Justin's lifelong sentence.

How often would Justin have to face situations like this?

Could he handle it?

Could I handle it?

Could our family handle it?

I was strong, so of course I could handle it.

Or maybe not.

I fooled myself into believing we would be alright. I put my emotions into a mental compartment, hoping the lid would stay on and keep the pain locked away. Little did I know stashing these feelings was like storing dynamite next to a lighter.

I thought about Justin's reasoning after the cross-country meet. We were not the only ones dealing with hard things. We knew this was happening not only to kids with Tourette Syndrome, but to many people who are different for reasons they cannot control. I know many parents of great kids who have brown or black skin. There are kids with medical conditions that make them walk or talk differently.

I gained a much deeper understanding of parent worry. Knowing we were not alone was a comfort—but only to an extent. Being together wouldn't take away the fact that the safety of our children was at risk.

I told myself I could not let situations like this paralyze me and control my behavior. I would do my part with our family in our little corner of the world to keep fighting to make things better.

However, these ideas and feelings would have to wait, because Justin had more travel coming up and I had to plan.

CHAPTER 28

Camp Twitch and Shout!

When the July after eighth grade finally arrived, Justin packed all by himself. The camp was organized and provided the kids with a list of everything to bring. This was perfect for Justin. He took the list and laid everything out and checked off every item.

With his suitcase packed, we headed to the airport. Ron and I got special passes to go to the airport gate with him so we could put him into the hands of the flight attendant. Someone from camp would be waiting for him at the gate in Atlanta.

Justin had been on planes before, but this would be his first solo flight. He was nervous about going alone, but he was even more excited to get to camp. When emotions run high for a kid with TS, the tics get worse.

As we walked into the airport and headed to security, Justin started tic'ing the word "bomb." *Not a great thing to do in an airport.* His physical tics were acting up, and he was basically a walking mess.

We nudged him to hand the security team one of his cards so he could explain that he did not in fact have a bomb.

Justin gave them the card, but the security team had a job to do. Any mention of a bomb had to be taken seriously, Tourette Syndrome or not. This was another moment where those darn verbal tics made life so difficult. Had Justin been twisting his head, no one would have reacted. But the word "bomb" in an airport…well that could not be ignored. The way this condition leads people to say the most inappropriate words at the perfect time is something comedians strive to achieve.

The security agents were serious and pulled us aside. They took the carry-on Justin was holding and asked for his checked bag to be removed from the belly of the plane. Both were searched for this bomb he was yelling about. We were quiet and cooperative. We knew we had no bomb, so it was best to simply let them do their thing.

There was no laughter in the moment of this situation.

Once everything was emptied out, they let us pack it all back up and we were off to the gate. We thanked them profusely because we were well aware this situation could have gone in many different directions. We knew there were a lot of "privileged" reasons we were not detained for questioning.

When we got to the gate, the flight attendant came out to meet us. Thankfully, the flight was not sold out, so to keep a better eye on Justin, they upgraded him to first class! He thought this was the greatest thing in the world. He strutted onto the plane like he owned the place. He handed his cards out to all the people sitting around him, and everyone was understanding.

Being at camp was an incredible experience. Not only did he get to meet Brad Cohen, but he got to meet the actor James Wolk, who played Brad in the movie. He reconnected with his buddies from YA training and made many new friends.

Camp Twitch and Shout was like any other camp—except when it wasn't. The kids went kayaking, paddleboarding, and did high ropes courses. They had a talent show and ate together in the mess hall. They told stories around the campfire. It was a week where they could all be themselves, surrounded by kids just like them. It was heaven. The kids would pick up each other's tics, and Justin would come home every year with a new repertoire of sounds and words to add to the chaos of Tourette Syndrome. Things were never quiet there—never a dull moment!

Justin attended Camp Twitch and Shout the next year as a camper and the following year as a Counselor in Training (CIT). Since then, he has donated his time every year as a counselor. He says there is nothing more rewarding, and at age 22, he still looks forward to camp as his favorite week of the year. He sees his younger self in the campers and does everything in his power to let these kids know that the only limits they have are the ones they impose on themselves.

I'll never forget the first time Justin came home from camp. He was a new kid. Being with his "people" in an environment where he could openly be himself was the best medicine. It was a week with nothing to hold back, where he could fully relax and have fun.

Camp was the perfect antidote after the difficulty of the eighth-grade-trip roommate situation, the visit to the museum, and being stopped in in the airport because of his tics. He would need these experiences to get him through some really tough tics that were about to unexpectedly enter his life in a debilitating fashion.

CHAPTER 29

Norway

All at once, a lot of different things started happening for Justin. A few days after he left for the eighth-grade DC trip, we received an email from the National Tourette Syndrome Association. It announced that the Tourette Syndrome Association of Norway had received a grant that would provide an all-expenses-paid trip for seven Youth Ambassadors from the US to travel for a cross-cultural exchange experience with students from Norway and Hungary.

Justin was thrilled about this opportunity. He applied and felt lucky to be selected. The trip would take place only a few weeks after Justin's return from camp Twitch and Shout.

Things got even better a month before he was set to go. One of the male chaperones had to cancel, and Ron was invited to take his place. He didn't have to deliberate long before accepting the offer!

I became the coordinator for the group of six other students who would be meeting at Newark Airport in New Jersey. They all came from different states, but luckily, Justin knew a few of them from our prior conferences and his experiences at camp.

Sadly, three days before the trip, a horrible crime was committed in Norway. This was very unusual, because Norway is a country with one of the lowest crime rates in the world. A lone person detonated several bombs in government buildings in the capital city, which is where our group would be traveling. He then went to the island of Utøya disguised as a security officer and shot and killed more than sixty people—mostly children—in what would become the worst tragedy in Norway's history.

The US government immediately imposed a "no fly" order, meaning the trip was in jeopardy. At this point, they knew little about the perpetrator and had to confirm it was not an act of terrorism.

Thankfully, the day before the trip, the ban was lifted, and the kids would be allowed to travel.

This became the adventure of a lifetime for Justin and Ron. The day after our kids were to arrive, there would be a large memorial event for those who had perished. I reached out to all the families, and the kids opted to bring teddy bears they could leave at the site as a show of support.

When Ron and Justin returned home, they described the impact of this portion of the trip. They felt a profound sadness; however, they were so inspired to see how people came together to support one another. They saw people leaning on each other to cry. Strangers were hugging strangers simply to show a kindness.

While it's difficult to define a tragic event as inspiring, it taught all of us a powerful lesson about the need to comfort others—and that sometimes, being there says far more than words ever could.

Ron and Justin recalled the raw emotions they felt. Everyone on the trip bonded. They will always remember the bonding. All of the kids had Tourette Syndrome—so different in culture, yet they were so alike. It was a chance for them to sightsee, hike, and to just be themselves. They made friendships that still exist today.

There was another milestone for Justin on this trip. He had his first kiss! Throughout the trip, he grew close with a girl. She had fears about participating in some of the activities, and Justin was there to support her. Ron saw a new side of Justin's compassion for others—it was so heartening and adorable to see our child, with limited social skills, know just what to do to comfort another person.

____

CHAPTER 30

Life in a Wheelchair

Although the Norway trip was wonderful, the hiking was brutal on Justin's ankles. They were not in great shape before the trip because of tics, so we had Justin outfitted with braces ahead of time. Now Justin was starting high school, which was a big change that brought lots of nerves and anxiety. Add Tourette Syndrome to the mix, and it's the perfect storm for difficulty.

This difficulty came in the form of increased ankle tics but also brought us something new. Justin developed a tic in his hip that looked like the crane kick delivered by the Karate Kid. His leg did everything but fly into the air.

We all scrambled to get out of the way when this tic came, because no one wanted to be the recipient of its violent blow. Trips to the emergency room were becoming common. These kicking tics were horribly painful and prone to causing either a fracture or dislocation.

Justin got new braces for his ankles, and he used his old friend Herman the Cane to help him balance.

The week he started high school, Konnor started college. Thankfully, Stefanye was starting her senior year at college, so she had an apartment and didn't need move-in help.

Ron and I had a difficult decision to make. We knew there was no way both of us could take Konnor to school. Justin needed one of us to be with him—his tics were simply too difficult and violent for us to leave him with anyone else.

We decided that Ron would take Konnor and I would stay home. Although I agreed with this decision, having to miss the college drop-off was so hard. Konnor was good about it, and if he didn't understand or was angry, he never showed it.

I felt so guilty. We packed up the car, I gave him huge hugs, the typical motherly advice, and watched them drive off. I sat in the driveway and cried my eyes out for about half an hour. But then, I dusted off and told myself to be excited for our first visit to Storrs, Connecticut, to come later in the year.

After about a week of school, it was obvious that Herman the cane was no help. Justin could barely walk. I took him to the doctor, where we got difficult news.

He had sprained both ankles, and the muscles in his right hip had separated from the ligaments, reducing his range of motion by 80%.

Walking was out of the question. Justin would have to use a wheelchair.

This brought another dimension to our lives. We had no idea how to navigate life with a wheelchair. There were more questions than answers.

We were going to have to look really hard for the silver linings.

This happened to be the day of the school's first football game—the first time Justin was supposed to march in the school's marching band. Obviously, that wasn't going to happen—but he wanted to play and support the band. As we drove to pick up the wheelchair, I called the school and spoke to one of the band directors to let him know I wanted to follow the bus with Justin and the wheelchair so he could go to the game.

The director said he would have no part of that.

Uh-oh.

Then he kindly explained to me that Justin was part of the band family, and they would figure it out. Justin would be helped on and off the bus by other band members, and the chair would go on the equipment bus. If Justin struggled to "wheel" it, a band member would be made available to push him.

The director would have it no other way.

Wow.

I cried tears of disbelief. Total joy. Justin was even more thrilled.

What I didn't know was the three band directors had called everyone together to let them know a family member needed their help. They instructed the more than 250 kids to be on the lookout for Justin and that it was their responsibility to help him when he needed it. Most important, they were to treat him as they always had and ensure that he was always included.

And did they ever!

These kids were amazing. Throughout the entire season and beyond, they were always there when Justin needed help.

What made it even more special was that the directors never told us they did this. In their minds, it was what needed to be done. We found out from one of the students who had been especially helpful to Justin. Although Ron, Justin, and I have thanked every member of that band (and especially the directors) repeatedly, they will never know the magnitude of our gratitude.

One problem solved, and on the to the next....

The physical therapist who set Justin up with his wheelchair was wonderful. He showed us everything. Wheelchairs have a lot of moving parts—I felt like there were a million levers! He showed us how Justin would get in and out of the chair. He showed us how to use crutches for support, so he didn't put weight on either leg as he shifted from the chair to a different seat.

He showed me how to fold up the chair to get it into the back of my SUV. That thing was heavy! I needed to eat more Wheaties!

Next problem.

Our house was not wheelchair accessible. I knew Justin could navigate the first and second floors. But how was I going to get him out of the car and into the house? We had three stairs in the garage leading up to the house.

As we pulled into the garage, Justin and I looked at each other. I immediately said, "What the fuck are we going to do?" And then we started laughing. We realized laughing would be better than crying.

We put our heads together and figured it out. I got the chair and wheeled him up to the steps. I got out the cane, and he used the cane for support on one side and me on the other. Between his arm strength and me, he made it up the stairs without using his legs.

Thankfully, we had a bench right by the door, so I sat Justin down on it, then—with all my brute strength—I lifted the chair up the steps and transferred him to it. I was red faced and huffing and puffing!

That little two-minute drill left us exhausted, but we knew it was one we needed to get used to—we would be doing it for months to come.

The saddest part was realizing how many places were not wheelchair accessible. We were invited to an event where there would be a ceremony in the upstairs part of the building and the reception was downstairs. Upon arrival, we learned there was no elevator.

Ron carried Justin up the stairs, sat him down, then went and got the wheelchair. No more than five minutes later, Justin announced that he needed to go to the bathroom. Normally, this would not be a problem, but since the only bathroom in the building was on the first floor, we had to make another tiring trip down and back up the steps.

Unfortunately, these types of things happened more than they should have. It is amazing how you never think about walking up a few steps to get into a building or someone's home. All of these became challenges.

Justin accepted this plight really well. He had an amazing attitude, always seemed happy, and never once complained. Not once.

In fact, the situation helped build his social skills. For the first time, he was the center of attention without having to act out with bad behavior. People wanted to help him. And he soaked it up. He learned to roll the chair really fast, and—much to my extreme fear—he learned to do wheelies! I was petrified he would tip over backward. Although I didn't know it at the time, years later, Justin told me he fell several times, but there was always someone to pick him back up. Somehow Justin was using all the social skills he'd learned from Mary to his advantage and was taking people up on their offers of help. He found a way to make the most out of a difficult situation.

────

CHAPTER 31

My Son, the Sideshow

Justin didn't consider long-term repercussions—that was my job.

I was scared. Really scared. Where was this going to lead?

I'd put a lid on my feelings after Justin's school trip, but—compounded by the wheelchair—my emotions were brewing.

The only thing keeping the explosion from happening was my fear of being vulnerable. Years ago, when Justin was on suicide watch, I'd attempted to share my feelings, pains, and frustrations with friends, but the result had been dismissal, and Ron and I felt we'd been left to fend for ourselves.

I'd been abandoned by people I thought were my friends.

I was petrified of sharing anything with anyone. I did everything I could to push the feelings inside. I kept pushing…

…until I couldn't.

I was terrified Justin would never walk again. The tics were showing no signs of letting up, and I became concerned that the longer he went without walking, the more atrophied his muscles would be.

I was conflicted. On one hand, Justin seemed so happy. People were helping him, and he had been accepted into the marching-band family. On the other hand, he was not getting calls to go out and do things, and nobody was coming over to hang out with him. His only interactions with friends were when we made plans with other families.

His social skills were much better, but when you live in the same city and go through school with the same kids, your past has a way of sticking with you. If this bothered Justin, he didn't say anything—maybe he didn't realize he *could* have more of a social life. Maybe he didn't know what he was missing.

But I did.

I made excuses. I assumed no one called because of the difficulties his wheelchair presented. It was tricky to navigate, and you had to plan. What kid wanted to commit to that level of planning?

But I was willing to plan! If only the phone would ring for Justin and someone would ask me to plan an outing. But kids don't do that kind of thing. If only one person had called Justin to say, "Hey, we're going to the basketball game, want to come?" Ron and I would have made it happen.

But they didn't.

We had become friendly with a great group of marching-band parents, and we all sat together in the stands during the football games. They would happily point out their kids on the field, and although I enjoyed seeing them, I missed being able to point out mine. Justin sat in his chair on the sidelines. He played his instrument, but it wasn't the same.

Often, the conversation would focus on Justin's tics. They were funny and even brought comedic relief. During a practice, the band director was yelling at the girls on the dance team and at the exact right moment, Justin tic'ed the phrase "bitches and hoes." It brought everyone to hysterical laughter!

But there was a tough side to this.

Couldn't anyone see the heartbreaking side and acknowledge it? I wished someone had pulled me aside to say, "I know we are all laughing, but Lisa, are you okay?"

Didn't anyone consider for even one moment that their laughter at his condition made me wonder if it would be the only part of Justin that people connected to? Was he purely the entertainment?

I was willing to bet other people would see it differently if they had to walk in Justin's shoes. Could they handle a single day screaming "Penis!" at the top of their lungs, dropping the word "fuck" in the synagogue, and yelling the N-word with no ability to stop?

How could friends only focus on the funny and not realize how hard it was for Justin to go through all of this?

Justin's favorite band was Rush. They were scheduled to play in Cleveland right before the start of Justin's ninth grade year, and Ron got tickets for the two of them to go and have a wonderful father-and-son experience. They made it about ten minutes before Justin began tic'ing so badly they had to leave. We didn't realize the strobe lights in the concert would stimulate tics.

It nearly killed me when this happened.

How I wished someone would have asked, "How was the concert?" and when I told them, they could have said, "That must be so hard."

But these things didn't happen.

Justin went to the high school's homecoming dance, where the DJ had a light show. Not long after he got there, Justin called us to pick him up. Many of my friends knew he left, but no one said a word.

Would our son be able to enjoy anything?

Even though it seemed funny on the outside, I wished people would see the reality of this hardship.

And how could they not see this worry was paralyzing me?

I found myself surrounded by a crowd of people yet feeling totally alone. I wished with all my heart that one of them would see beyond the brave face I wore and recognize my stress.

I often found myself being quiet, lost in my own headspace.

I had my sister friends I'd met at the conference, but for some reason, I didn't use their lifeline. They were not in town to "see" me, and it didn't occur to me they might be feeling the same things.

Because I was so afraid of being a burden to my friends, when I found myself in that quiet place, I'd force myself snap out of it and put on my happy face and pretend. The easiest way to pretend was to tell myself that other people came first. I deflected. I did my best to focus on their kids, ask them how they were doing—if I made them feel important, then maybe at some point, they would find a way to focus on me.

I was certain being strong was what they would admire about me.

After all, when people deal with major illnesses, everyone talks about admiring their strength.

Being strong is exhausting.

Every day, I put on my makeup to look pretty. Then came the imaginary superhero cape I'd put on too—the one that hid the person I didn't want anyone to see.

Our family had been through so much—life and death—and I'd handled it.

We went through the loss of friends, and I'd handled it.

We received a diagnosis of a lifelong medical condition…and I'd handled it.

I was sick of handling it.

I didn't want to lose friends again.

Watching Justin—who had to find so much strength just to exist—have setbacks tore me apart from the inside; I was afraid to share it with anyone.

This setback felt different—out of my control. I told myself to just get through the day.

I was spiraling into a dark, desolate place where my loneliness grew into anger.

By the end of every day, I was so stressed, I would completely fall apart. In secret.

I sobbed, but nobody knew.

In fact, until I wrote this chapter of the book, no one—not Ron, not Justin, not Stefanye or Konnor—knew how I felt. They had no idea I secretly cried in the bathroom every night after everyone had fallen asleep. I would talk myself into so much worry that I'd explode into tears that no one saw.

I so desperately needed someone to see how exhausted I was and to offer something—any kind of empathy, a shoulder to cry on.

Because that is what I would have done.

Tell me I look like shit—please. Do it in a nice way, of course—no, maybe I need to be hit over the head with it.

Watch me struggle to lift that 800-pound gorilla of a wheelchair into my trunk and say, "Let me help you with that."

So many moms and dads in the school pick-up line sat by and watched. No one ever came to help me.

Because that is what I would have done.

I assumed being the superhero was what others liked about me.

I subconsciously believed I deserved nothing and that everyone else deserved my full attention.

And when they didn't reciprocate, I felt so hurt and sad that it turned to anger.

But at the same time, I was fearful of losing them. I was a hot mess.

It's no wonder I didn't get what I wanted—what I needed.

How could anyone possibly know?

I was standing with my back to the crowd—yelling at the wall and wondering why I was alone—when all I needed to do was turn around.

It wasn't until a few years later that I would process all this. My friend Linda had the courage to say something.

"Lisa, I've never seen you cry."

At first, I wasn't sure how to handle her concern.

Why was this important?

I told her I'd grown up being taught that crying was a sign of weakness.

I told her no one likes someone weak.

She corrected me.

The gift of hindsight has helped me see that the giant wall I built didn't let anyone come to the other side. I was my own worst enemy. If I'd allowed myself to be vulnerable, I could have eased some of my anguish.

I unfairly assumed my new friends would be just like the others, but that was wrong.

Linda taught me something important that day—and for that, I'm so thankful.

She said I didn't need to carry the entire burden. She helped me understand that asking for support or asking someone to listen did not equal complaining. And, if it did come off as complaining, I had every right to do so. I was in pain—I was entitled to blow up, lose it, or do whatever I needed to allow others to help me.

I deserved grace and compassion.

It's called being human.

Linda also told me that the right people, good friends, enjoy being there for someone else. They like to feel needed, and I tended to push everyone away without knowing it.

Perhaps I could have said to one person, "Can you help me?" It sounds and feels strange, it was so hard to utter those words.

I was the caregiver. I was supposed to take care of everyone else, no one was supposed to take care of me.

Wrong.

I'm ashamed that I hid my feelings from my husband and my family. They were—still are—my biggest fans, cheerleaders, confidantes. Hiding things from them was a mistake. These are people who would never judge me and would support me above doing anything else. If only I'd seen that.

I learned I didn't need to take the blame either. The people around me could have done more. Now I see things from multiple angles.

I didn't love myself. I was devaluing myself by putting everyone in front of me. What I didn't realize was that not loving yourself sends out a vibe. I was sending out an unconscious message to stay away.

This is still a struggle for me. I still feel the need to control my emotions, and I have the tendency to put others first. But now I recognize it, and I am working toward this personal improvement.

I recently started working with a new coach named Libby, who has me doing an exercise I highly recommend. It's so easy for me to tell my husband and my kids that I love them, so Libby has me look in the mirror at least once each day and tell me I love myself. It feels awkward, but it's important. The idea is that if I tell myself often enough, I'll start to believe it. Believing it will lead to feeling better on the inside, which will let me show a much better side of me to the world.

—————

CHAPTER 32

A Wrinkle-Free Solution

As Justin's ninth grade year in the wheelchair went on, we saw no signs of improvement and landed right back in the maze.

Thanksgiving, Hanukkah, Christmas, New Year's—all in the wheelchair.

Spring break—in the wheelchair.

Every visit to the doctor brought absolutely no encouragement. We were told to simply hope the tic moved on.

Hope.

This felt so passive.

My fear that Justin would never walk again was looking more and more likely. I could physically see the loss of strength and muscle mass.

I knew there were kids with Tourette Syndrome who had permanent injuries or unfixable situations, but Ron and I refused to believe this would be the outcome for our son.

He would walk again—he *had* to walk again—even if it meant hitting more walls, we would have to keep looking.

I needed to snap out of my self-imposed gloom and get back with the program and find a solution. After all, problem-solving was my specialty.

Energy diverted.

Although we loved our neurologist, he was in his eighties and partially retired. Because Justin was a longstanding patient, he took our appointments, but I began to question whether he was the right doctor for us, so we opted to make a change.

We asked people for names of new doctors, and our next gift came from an unlikely source.

I was introduced to a new friend, and we met for coffee. We talked about her son's struggles with a disability that impacted his ability to walk, and I opened up about our story. After letting her know the type of help we needed, she said she had our answer—her ex-husband.

As soon as she said that, my mind went in a million directions. How could I ask her to request a favor, knowing they were not on good terms? But she was willing to make a call for us and got us an appointment the next day—which was incredible, and I'm still thankful for this gift.

Her ex-husband was a doctor. He didn't specialize in Tourette Syndrome, but he had access to plenty of resources and felt confident he could help. He spent almost two hours with us and asked Justin a million questions. He videotaped Justin's tics so he could send it to a colleague in another state to get an opinion. He exposed Justin to different scenarios that helped us identify things that triggered tics. We never put two and two together, but that's when we learned flashing lights were a huge trigger.

The doctor also explained that Justin had a rare form of tics called dystonic tics. These involve the large muscle groups and can be incredibly painful. They have the power to break bones and braces. They were the reason he had that awful tic in his leg and hip.

Things were starting to make sense.

The doctor gave us some great information. He made no promises but told us he would be our new quarterback and would be there with us to figure out anything and everything we could.

We walked out of his office with a plan. His assistant became my new best friend. Thank goodness for Fran! She scheduled all our appointments and told us where to go on what days.

Every test came back negative, which was good, but also frustrating because we still didn't have answers.

Until we met Dr. Micah Baird, physiatrist—not psychiatrist—*physiatrist*. I had never heard of this specialty, but it focuses on pain management and reduction.

Thank goodness for Ron, who can find humor in so many things. He was my rock, and he carried this appointment. It was fun! How wild is that? We laughed in a therapeutic way. Ron jumped right in with the craziness of Justin's tics. As Dr. Baird listened, he stood by the examination table near Justin's legs. Suddenly, I realized the karate kick was about to happen.

I jumped up and yelled, *"Get out of the way!"*

He was about to get a swift kick to the face.

Dr. Baird had this look of total astonishment, paused, then said, "I've never seen anything like *that* before."

Suddenly we were all laughing, yet serious at the same time.

Dr. Baird went on to say, "I'm hooked. I can't make promises, but I can make it my mission to help you."

I stood up and clapped. I wanted to hug him but felt it would be inappropriate.

Dr. Baird told us he needed to do some research. There was a lot of work being done at Yale University, and he wanted to reach out to them. He needed a few weeks to investigate some possible solutions, then we would all get back together.

He delivered! When we had our second appointment, Dr. Baird suggested we try Botox. He explained that in the typical usage, the injections block certain chemical signals from nerves, mostly signals that cause muscles to contract. The most popular use of these injections was to temporarily relax facial muscles that cause wrinkles on the forehead and around the eyes.

In Justin's case, Dr. Baird would surgically inject Botox at the point where the nerves met the muscles in hopes of blocking the tic signal from the brain. The tic/brain signal would likely move to another place, but the goal was to free up the hip and leg to stop tic'ing and allow Justin to heal and walk again.

Justin would need to be under anesthesia, and the process would involve sending electrical impulses to help the doctors determine exactly which nerves and muscles were involved in this tic. When they identified them, they would zap in the Botox.

Of course, there were no promises, no guarantees, but Dr. Baird seemed confident there was a good chance of this working.

Surgery was scheduled for a week later. It would be a simple outpatient procedure, and Dr. Baird hoped we would see immediate results.

We did. The tic stopped.

We felt like a miracle had been achieved.

But nothing comes easy.

Justin returned to school the day after the procedure. In hindsight, we should have kept him home, but he woke up feeling okay, so off he went.

A few hours later, the school called to tell me Justin was in the nurse's office because he was having trouble breathing. The minute I got to school and saw him, I knew something was terribly wrong.

Thankfully, it was a three-minute drive from the school to our home.

The car ride was awful. I watched him struggle to breath and start to panic. The minute we got home, I called 911.

The paramedics were wonderful. I explained that he had just had surgery and wasn't sure if this was something left over from the anesthesia or if this was the tic moving to a new place. They listened to him and decided it would be best to get to the hospital as quickly as possible. They gave him oxygen, but we could physically see his chest heaving.

Stefanye was home for the weekend, so she called Ron.

I rode in the ambulance with Ron following in the car. Because they were monitoring Justin closely, I had to ride in the front seat so the paramedics could be right on top of my son. I was holding my breath because I was so scared that he might stop breathing. This was probably the scariest ride of my life. What made it even more frightening was the number of cars that didn't stop, move to the side, slow down, or do *anything* to make way for the ambulance—sirens blaring. The driver had trouble making the left turn out of our development! I was in shock.

I will jump on my soapbox and insist that if you hear an ambulance with sirens blaring, lights flashing, or both: please, please, pull over to the side of the road. If you were riding in the back of that vehicle in any kind of an urgent situation—believe me, you would want others to move for you.

When we arrived at the hospital, the ER doctors immediately assumed Justin was having a panic attack. We told them about his Tourette Syndrome, and as expected, they told us they were "familiar" with Tourette's but insisted this was a panic attack.

Clearly, they did not know as much as they should have, and they treated us quite poorly. They were unwilling to listen to anything we had to say. Our explanations of the years we'd spent dealing with TS fell on deaf ears.

Because we knew it was necessary to calm Justin down, we agreed to a dose of anti-anxiety medication. Whenever someone can't breathe, it leads to panic, and getting a handle on the panic was essential. Besides, one dose wouldn't hurt him.

The drugs they administered relaxed Justin and allowed him to sleep.

We realized this was a tic, and we wondered how long it would be hanging around.

As we figured, the tic persisted. But because we knew it was a tic, Justin was able to manage his breathing. This helped ease the anxiety, and we opted not to continue the anxiety medication.

But something strange happened. Because the tic was painful around Justin's ribs, he asked Ron to lift him up to crack his back. When Ron did this, the tic stopped. Whatever Ron did, it moved the diaphragm into a position that made the tic go away.

Phew—crisis over.

About a week after the Botox surgery, we took Justin to physical therapy so he could learn to walk again, and we hit another wall.

The therapist we worked with was wonderful, but he said the bursitis in Justin's hip was so bad that we needed to see an orthopedic doctor before he could help us. Justin would need to undergo one more surgical procedure to repair the damage from the tic.

Again, this was outpatient surgery, but we did talk with the anesthesiologist about the breathing tic that erupted after the last surgery. He altered his plan and, thankfully, Justin was in and out.

He needed a bit more recovery time, but the minute we were allowed to take him back to PT, we were there.

It was a long process to get his muscles moving and strong enough to hold his weight. Justin was diligent about doing the exercises he was told to do, and Ron and I learned some massage techniques so we could get the blood flowing and keep the muscles from tightening up too much.

It took Justin a little over two months, but he finally stood up and started taking steps! I took a video of those first few steps, and I still cry when I watch him walk again.

Although we were scared, we never gave up. We knew the tics could come back, but we had a path forward. Justin would require two more Botox treatments in the next two years. Thank goodness for the amazing Dr. Baird!

CHAPTER 33

Becoming a Speaker

After the success of Justin's first Tolerance Fair, we started receiving requests for him to speak at a variety of events. Because we were constantly in and out of the ER, we had to decline many of them. He was able to speak before the Solon Rotary and for the current class of his "Dream Team" fifth grade teachers, but we kept it very low key.

Once Justin had made progress in physical therapy and was beginning to walk again, he felt ready for more speaking engagements, and he accepted a request from Beachwood Middle School. The principal reached out and asked if Justin would not only do a teacher presentation but wanted him to do a full school assembly! This was big! A full school assembly. *Wow.* Of course, Justin immediately agreed. He was still in the wheelchair, but the stage was accessible.

He rolled on stage and introduced himself as a student similar to all of them. He talked about playing in the band and made a joke about running on the cross-country team that got a huge laugh. The student response was all Justin needed to jumpstart his adrenaline.

Then he brought up how he was different.

Justin described his Tourette Syndrome and shared stories of how he was bullied and the way that made him feel. The room got quiet; the students paid attention. There were giant belly laughs when Justin described his adventure of tic'ing the bomb at the airport.

I stood in the back, in the dark, and cried quiet tears—which, of course, I hid. But these were not tears of sadness. These tears sprang from pure joy.

Toward the end of his speech, Justin described his time in the wheelchair and joked about his newfound wrinkle-free skin thanks to his Botox procedure. The students continued to laugh!

Then, he created a big moment. He told the students he had been in that chair for almost the entire school year, but he always kept the faith that he would walk again.

Then, he paused.

He looked down and said, "Give me a minute."

He paused again.

Slowly…very slowly…he stood up.

Justin gingerly walked across the stage with the microphone in his hand. Quietly, but with enough force so the students could hear it, he said, "Never give up."

The kids went wild and immediately rose to their feet!

And a speaking career was born.

———

CHAPTER 34

The Call

Three weeks after Justin's speech, and thirteen months after the Tolerance Fair, I got a call that changed everything.

"Hi, Lisa. You won't remember me, but I remember you. I came to the Tolerance Fair, and I am calling to let you know it changed our lives."

"Oh, my goodness—that is so kind of you."

"My daughter was despondent, and I didn't know how to help her. I saw a story on the news about your son and knew I needed to come to the event. I drove an hour to get there. I was desperate and would do anything for my daughter. While I was there, I connected with the Suicide Prevention Education Alliance. Their counselors got my daughter into a youth group, they gave us names of therapists, and now, she is a new person. She is still in treatment, but thanks to your event, she is happy and on the right path."

This woman and I chatted for a few more minutes, and we cried happy tears together. I let her know she'd rendered me speechless, which doesn't happen very often.

As soon as Justin got home from school, I shared every detail of the call with him. He was quiet for a few minutes, as he took in the enormity of the conversation. I could tell that all the events—the ups and downs of the last few months—were rushing through his mind.

Gradually, a huge smile lit up his face.

He looked at me and said, "Mom, we need to do this again."

CHAPTER 35

Honor Good Deeds

Justin was entering the tenth grade, and we could see such a difference in so many things about him. He had gained a beautiful sense of confidence. He had a way of walking into a room and lighting it up. He had a way of making people feel comfortable, and he exuded a sense of natural leadership wherever he went.

He had energy and it was contagious!

He had moved from "that awful kid" to a role model parents wanted their kids to be around.

Justin did an amazing job with the first Tolerance Fair, and his leadership and can-do attitude flourished as we started planning our next event.

Although the first Tolerance Fair was successful, we learned a lot about how we could make the next one better. Our goal—bigger, better, help more people! We would need a formal nonprofit organization, and that's how Honor Good Deeds was born.

At the first fair, we'd had forty-eight exhibitors. We sat down at our kitchen table and together decided we wanted to double that and shoot for a hundred exhibitors. We did some rough estimating on costs and determined we would need between $50,000 and $75,000 to hold the event. The number felt overwhelmingly high, and daunting, but we had faith and knew we could get there with hard work and creativity.

Although we felt challenged, we never thought about making things smaller. We had confidence in our abilities to pull it off. We marched forward knowing we were going to make mistakes and that in some cases, we would need to change our plan. After all, making mistakes was how we learned.

Of course, there were the naysayers—those who said there was no way we could raise the money. They were entitled to their opinions, but we knew we could do it. We could not let other people shatter our dreams. The words of that mom who told me we made a difference in her daughter's life thwarted anyone who doubted that we could accomplish this goal.

We were sad we couldn't hold the event in Solon—the place where it began. But we needed to find a new place because the Solon Recreation Center was too small for our big dreams!

More important, Mayor Drucker had been so supportive, we didn't want to leave her behind. Loyalty to someone who clearly stepped up for us was important. To deal with this, we came up with an idea: the Mayor's Challenge. Justin called Mayor Drucker and asked if she would lead this initiative. It would involve contacting every mayor in Northeast Ohio and asking them to proclaim the date of the fair as a day of tolerance in their city. We also asked Mayor Drucker to be the lead speaker to kick off the event.

She immediately agreed, wrote letters to all the mayors, and the proclamations began rolling in! Seventeen out of a thirty-seven cities agreed to participate—including every one of the largest areas surrounding Cleveland, which was perfect.

Because of all the therapy he had done, Justin was an expert at talking with adults. In his early years, he negotiated everything—every little thing—which helped him hone some darn good powers of persuasion. Something good came from that difficult childhood. This came in handy as we started to raise money.

Because of my event-planning business, I had a number of contacts throughout the city, and I had done business with all the major banks. I had recently met an executive who happened to have a child with a mild case of Tourette Syndrome. I told her our story—and that we were planning the next Tolerance Fair—and asked if she would meet with Justin. She agreed, and Justin immediately got to work on a PowerPoint presentation promoting various levels of sponsorship. We were hoping her company would donate $1,000, so we knew we had to ask for more. But how much?

We were a small, new organization with a proven reputation of only one event. To raise $50,000 to $75,000, we needed a lot of small donations or a few larger ones. Ron brought up his favorite quote, "Pigs get fat, hogs get slaughtered." We decided to ask for $5,000. The worst that could happen was that she'd say no, then we could adjust our strategy.

Justin, Ron, and I met with her at a Panera restaurant. After the introductions, fifteen-year-old Justin dove in with his presentation. He did all the talking, and Ron and I sat by and watched. He got about halfway through when the woman from the bank stopped him and said, "I'm in, how much do you need?" Justin skipped to the end and asked for $5,000, and she said, "Count me in, five thousand it is."

What just happened?

There was no negotiating.

She said she would give the entire thing!

Did we hear her correctly?

This was way too easy!

Ron, Justin, and I shared a silent communication to remain calm and wait until we got home to cheer and do cartwheels.

We had been so accustomed to bad things. It was time to let ourselves believe that good could happen. We deserved good things.

CHAPTER 36

Business Cards, Not the Sympathy Card

If you have ever seen the television show *Family Ties*, you're about to recognize that we were now living with Alex P. Keaton—a funny character who was a highly professional adult in a teenage body.

Justin enjoyed dressing up in suits, and he wore them to school. He didn't care if anyone criticized him. He was doing his thing, and he didn't sweat the small stuff. He was developing a humble confidence.

He still wasn't getting calls to go to the basketball game or the movies, but it never seemed to bother him. Although it was hard, Ron and I couldn't let it bother us either. Justin was doing the things gave him confidence and made him happy. We had to follow his lead and trust that he was doing what was right for him, even if it didn't fit our picture of what should be. On any given Friday night, instead of being out with friends, he was building his dream—his nonprofit. He created PowerPoints, made videos, and did a podcast.

To plan the next Tolerance Fair, Justin worked the phones like a pro. Ron and I became his transportation to many meetings where the executives could not turn down an ask from this tic'ing young entrepreneur.

And, yes—Justin did tic, and we never hid the fact that he had Tourette Syndrome. He shared his story, but we *never* played the sympathy card. Justin would be matter-of-fact in explaining his condition so people knew what to expect, then he moved on.

We were confident that nothing was ever offered because people felt sorry for Justin. Every meeting was completed with the utmost professionalism. He was well prepared and carried himself with confidence. There was no pity—only respect.

He designed his business card—he was so proud when they arrived!

Justin was never a shy kid, and he was always a talker. Putting these skills together, he figured out how to network. He had a firm handshake, and after every meeting, he asked the person if they could suggest other contacts for him to call for all aspects of the fair—whether it be a nonprofit to exhibit or a potential funder.

It worked!

People began calling Justin to recommend executives to contact for donations. This was exactly what we needed.

As impressive as Justin was in these meetings, he was still a teenager with a disability, and he was disorganized. Without realizing it, he and I had formed a business relationship. He ran the show, and I'd be behind the scenes helping him stay organized. Every executive needs a good assistant—that was me!

When we were in business mode, we acted like it. He would call me Lisa instead of Mom. Others found it funny, and it *was* amusing, but it didn't faze us. We slipped into an easy division of mom and co-worker.

Watching Justin work became pure joy.

One of the nonprofits that exhibited at the first fair invited us to attend their yearly gala. The minute we arrived, Justin left Ron and me to go work the room. He walked over to a man who was standing by himself and said, "Hi, you look like you need someone to talk with."

As luck would have it, the man happened to be the CEO of one of the banks in town. Justin started the conversation by asking what brought him to the event, and things progressed from there. Later in the evening, the CEO came up to Ron and me to tell us how impressed he was with Justin—his maturity and ease in conversation. He said he felt like Justin cared about him, and only when he asked did Justin tell his story.

There were many things I learned by watching our son network. For years, I avoided going to events where I didn't know anyone. Nothing was more terrifying than walking into a room filled with strangers, and I made matters worse by assuming everyone knew each other.

But watching Justin made me appreciate that I had missed out on meeting some cool people. I tried to figure out what was causing my hesitation, and I realized I didn't want to be rejected or look dumb for not knowing what to say.

I've read all kinds of articles and that recommend "starting lines" like "Tell me about you" or something that felt cheesy to me. By observing my son and experimenting on my own, I've learned it's best to just let conversation happen. I've approached people by introducing myself with a smile and an outstretched hand. I'll either mention something about the event and ask them how they feel about it, or I'll pay them a compliment. I've found that when I can get someone to talk about themselves, they are happy to engage.

I made a promise to myself that I would get better at this.

At this same event, the CEO of a company called Fairmount Minerals was being honored. The person who was introducing the award described the honoree, Chuck Fowler, as one of the most charitable people he knew. Their company lived by the motto, "Do good. Do well." And they not only talked the talk, they walked the walk!

During the introduction, the speaker issued a challenge to the students in the room—he told them that if they ever needed advice, Mr. Fowler was the type of person who would take their call.

Ron looked across the table at Justin and nodded his head. Justin called Mr. Fowler the next day. True to his reputation, Mr. Fowler took Justin's call. This began what would become a wonderful relationship—not only with Mr. Fowler, but with his entire family.

I'll never forget the first time we went to Mr. Fowler's office. He had photos of himself fishing with his grandchildren, and there was a giant fish on the wall—perfect opening! We had a lovely conversation, and he was all in.

The next day, I received an email from Mr. Fowler's daughter. Not only did she offer to help, but she sent a spreadsheet filled with organizations we could call to exhibit. She told us to use her name. We loved the initiative they took without being asked. They didn't say, "Let us know if we can help." They helped.

This was a lesson I had learned during our dark times. I appreciated the people who jumped in to do something—and I still do. I understand that not everyone knows what to do, but I've learned that when you really listen to what another person is going through, you can usually figure something out.

The events we attended, the networking, and the referrals really paid off. In the end, we raised $70,000, and the 2013 Tolerance Fair exceeded all our expectations! We welcomed 131 exhibitors and about 3,000 people attended.

This fair had some amazing highlights. First, we welcomed a well-known national speaker named Kyle Maynard. Kyle was born with no arms or legs and was the first person with no limbs to independently summit Mt. Kilimanjaro. He told a story of perseverance and self-acceptance that had people riveted.

But the most exciting and unforgettable part of the fair was an innovative idea Justin had to showcase diversity and how our differences bring us together: He created a surprise flash mob.

Flash mobs were being noticed a lot on social media, but there had not been a live one anywhere near where we lived. Justin worked with a friend to choreograph a simple dance—it looked complicated to me, but the kids seemed to catch on quickly. We quietly put out a call for teams of kids who would pay $10 to participate. The fee included the flash mob t-shirt, but our real motive was to ensure they would show up—they had to come that day to get the shirt.

We asked the team leaders to come to a rehearsal to learn the dance, and the leaders then taught it to their teams. We held several rehearsals to provide options, and the kids also did a video of the choreography so teams could refer to it as they learned. Either or both Ron and I attended the rehearsals to ensure there was adult supervision. One of the most memorable rehearsals was at the Cleveland Sight Center. We had a group of blind students mixed with sighted students who learned the dance together. It was magical.

On the day of the fair, the kids reported to a secret area behind some curtains. They came dressed in their clothes and were given their bright-orange flash mob t-shirts in the secret space. At the time we felt we had the most people in attendance, we cranked up the song "Born This Way" by Lady Gaga, and over a hundred kids ran out shouting and broke into the dance.

Watching the surprised expressions on the faces of attendees was awesome. Many got out their phones and started recording. Others joined in by dancing their own steps.

This is a life memory many of us will never forget.

We had kids of different skin colors, religions, sexualities, and abilities—Downs Syndrome kids, blind kids, kids in wheelchairs—who all came together to participate in this dance. Many of them knew the steps. Many didn't. It didn't matter—they all danced.

It is available at this link: https://www.youtube.com/watch?v=zYku Y6I-_ZM

There were not words sufficient to describe the novelty and meaning behind this flash mob that came together so perfectly. I often close my eyes, see it, and feel the joy in watching all these kids who didn't even know each other make something amazing happen.

This fair also featured many of the activities similar to those at the first one—but on a larger scale. Instead of a wheelchair obstacle course, we featured actual wheelchair basketball, soccer, and rugby games that ran throughout the day.

The Cleveland Sight Center provided a truly unique experience. They had blind people use their white canes to guide sighted people around the aisles of the event. It showcased the ability many people discount in people dealing with sight impairments.

Because we had so many exhibitors, we put together a program that people could take home as a resource. Each exhibiting organization had one page to showcase the three pillars of the fair—an overview of their target audience, the services they offer, and volunteer opportunities.

To further this message, we created an online directory from the program pages so anyone could come to our website for resources. We didn't charge the organizations a listing fee to ensure people would have access to anything our city had to offer. As time went on, this enabled organizations who were not able to exhibit at our fair to educate about their work.

We celebrated our success but immediately got to work on the next fair. We had to challenge ourselves because after doing this twice, we knew we needed to make it even bigger and better. We would need some new and creative ideas.

We realized that one of the most special things about the organization was that it was essentially run by a student—Justin. Why not get more teens involved? We created the Tolerance Fair Leadership Academy. Based on our experience, we knew how to create a large-scale event, and we were confident we could provide some incredible real-life experience to kids as they prepared for college. The program would run for nine months and would teach the students teamwork, goal setting, budgeting, fundraising, networking, contract negotiation, event planning, and much more. We formed partnerships with other nonprofits to train the students in topics such as interpersonal communications, writing skills, follow-up, and time management.

We sent flyers to ten schools, asking guidance counselors to recommend candidates for the Leadership Academy, and within a few weeks, we registered an amazing group of twenty-two students.

We did charge a fee for participation, which covered our costs for the training—but more important, we felt it would prompt the families to ensure their kids had skin in the game. We didn't want the parents to become involved in the details, but we needed them to be supportive. One of the great byproducts some of the parents mentioned was that it prompted some incredible parent-child conversations.

We kicked off the group with a weeklong training event that was mandatory. It ran Monday through Friday for two hours in the morning. It was fantastic! Not only did the kids bond with each other, but they bonded with us. It was an incredible group of kids who were highly motivated.

Each student participated at their own level. There was a core group of leaders who rose to the top and got the most out of the experience. Some did little, and that was okay—it was all part of the learning. Every student who wanted an opportunity to meet with a corporate executive got the chance to attend a fundraising meeting. They put on business attire and rode the elevators to top-floor board rooms.

The executives we met with were so impressed with the ability of the students. Ron and I rarely said a word—they ran it all. We were merely the transportation. It was so rewarding to listen in on the Skype calls they did with Justin to practice the things they wanted to say.

We were so thankful to these executives. Many had supported the fair financially in the past and it would have simply taken a phone call to renew their support. However, they recognized the experience we were providing the kids and were happy to meet with our students.

We challenged the students to be creative and make this fair bigger and better than the past two—a tall order because of the giant success we had in the past, but they delivered!

They created a campaign called Good Deeds Matter, which involved selling cardboard puzzle pieces for $1 each. The pieces were uniform in size to enable joining the pieces into mosaics. People who bought them were instructed to decorate the piece describing an act of kindness they had done. The goal was to create a visual representation of kindness and provide ideas to others on good deeds they could perform.

The kids did a great job in promoting this. Some asked their churches and temples to allow them to sell the pieces at a table after services. Others sold them in their grandparents' community homes and to their neighbors. Some students weren't comfortable with the sales aspect, and that was fine. That was the beauty of the leadership academy—there was something for everyone. Before the fair, we had several hundred mosaics, and even more pieces were decorated at the fair.

We welcomed back the Singing Fingers. One of their members was not able to attend due to illness and shortly after the fair, we received a call telling us she had died. We were so humbled and honored to learn that she wanted Justin to speak at her memorial service. Another group that had done a play for the 2014 fair called to tell us they wrote a play about Justin. We were in disbelief but felt so much gratitude that Justin's message was having this kind of an impact.

Like the other events, the 2014 Tolerance Fair was a great success. We welcomed 140 exhibitors and 4,000 people.

The feedback continued to roll in with stories of lives being changed. A few days after the fair, I dropped Justin off at school and noticed a girl walk up to him. They stopped to talk. Justin later told me that he didn't know her, but she had attended the fair and watched the flash mob. She told him she lived with anxiety and after seeing all the students having fun, she and her mom sought out a group to help her. She was excited to begin a new journey.

A few days later, we learned that a girl in marching band approached one of the organizations to share something she designed. She let us know that after seeing Justin navigate life in a wheelchair, she designed an inclusive picnic table that had benches and spaces for wheelchairs.

We were never short on stories motivating us to keep moving forward.

And the Winner Is...

There is an organization in Cleveland called the Maltz Museum of Jewish Heritage. It was one of our loyal exhibitors. They held an annual contest called Stop the Hate—funded by their founders, Milton and Tamar Maltz. Scholarship prizes were awarded to the winners with $40,000 granted to first place, $15,000 to second place and $10,000 to third place. Additionally, a $10,000 grant award was to be given to the school attended by the first place winner.

To enter, students submitted a 500-word essay about how they focused on stopping hate and making their community a better place. Volunteer readers selected the top ten essays, and the students were invited to read their essays at a large, well-attended event, where a panel of community leaders judged them.

Justin was very excited to enter. We felt he had a good chance of winning one of the top prizes. Thankfully, he had become a good writer and poured his passion out on the paper.

I still remember when the phone rang, and Justin was told he was a finalist. We were thrilled and nervous! All the student finalists had to attend a rehearsal where they read their essays for Mr. Maltz. Parents were not allowed to attend.

The event was held at Cleveland's Severance Hall, which is the home of the world-renowned Cleveland Orchestra. It is a beautiful building and carries a great deal of prestige—intimidating to a teenager hoping to win a big prize!

I sat in the lobby at Severance Hall waiting for Justin to finish the rehearsal. When he came out, he was white as a ghost. He told me that he had no chance of winning. He said each essay was better than the next.

Being supportive parents, we went through the drill of telling Justin he should be honored to simply be included in the group. If he won something, great, but if not, that would be just fine too. No matter what, we were so proud.

The night of the event, my stomach was a mess. Both Ron and I were so nervous for Justin. We knew some people in the audience, and we did our best to socialize.

As the event started, one by one, each student got up to read their essays. We were blown away by the professionalism and passion. Justin had been right. All the kids were incredible. Although I believed in our son, everyone on that stage deserved to win. I wanted Justin to win so badly, but I was fearful he would not.

By now, Justin had become an accomplished speaker. He never got nervous, but this night was different. As he was called to speak, he looked subdued. This was not like him. Before reading his speech, he would have to answer a special question from Mr. Maltz. As the question was read, we could see a smile coming to Justin's face—he knew the answer. He stepped to the podium, gave a heartfelt response, and read his essay.

He began: "September 18, 2010, is the day that changed my life forever. On that day, I went from living in the shadows to becoming a spokesperson for tolerance and acceptance..."

I felt like the evening was playing out in slow motion. When the last student finished reading, it was time to announce the winners. There was a break to allow the judges to tally their scores—which took only about ten minutes, but it felt like hours.

Mr. Maltz announced the third-place winner.

I prayed: *Please, not yet.*

Another student was named third-place winner.

Deep breath.

Mr. Maltz slowed things down and started chatting!

Does he not realize how hard my heart is pounding?

My knees were shaking.

I prayed again.

Please—not yet.

Mr. Maltz announced another name.

By this time, I was certain I was going to lose it. My heart was racing, and all I could think about was how thankful I was that I had not eaten much because I was sure I was going to be sick.

Mr. Maltz announced a drum roll.

Inside, I was screaming: *Just make the announcement!*

And then I heard it.

Mr. Maltz said, "And the winner is…"

(Insert a pause that lasted longer than forever.)

"Justin Bachman!"

Confetti fell from the ceiling and music played!

Ron and I sprang to our feet!

I sobbed tears of joy.

We clapped and hugged, and I don't know how, but Justin found us in the audience, and we made eye contact.

He had done it. After all his hard work, this was truly deserved.

They brought out a giant check and asked Justin to speak again. He was gracious in his acceptance. He complimented all the other students and was so genuine. There was a reception after the event, and everyone came up to congratulate us. It was a night we will never, ever forget. I can close my eyes at any moment and feel the pride and gratitude we experienced that night.

Shortly after that night, our phone rang. A tenth grader named Erin King was calling. I felt like I was talking with another Justin.

She had won a prize in the high school sophomore category. She was so impressed with our work and wanted to know if she could get involved. Not only did she get involved—she dove in with both feet. She became a part of our family and one of Justin's closest friends. We didn't know it at the time, but Erin would go on to lead our next Tolerance Fair Leadership Academy and help us move forward.

CHAPTER 38

Navigating the Speaking Circuit as a High School Student

After the incredible moment he had at Beachwood Middle School where he stood up and walked from his wheelchair—and after experiencing the applause—Justin announced that he would be launching a speaking program.

When Justin said something, it happened.

The principal at Beachwood made some recommendations to other schools, and before we knew it, the phone was ringing regularly with requests. We began posting on social media and sending emails to people we knew in education to get the word out.

Sadly, we received criticism from people who figured they knew what was best for us. They assumed we were forcing this on Justin and that I wrote his speeches.

Nope—never the case.

The choice to speak was Justin's and his alone. It was his passion. There was something about being on stage that ignited a fire in him. And he was good at it—really good at it. The rule we laid down was that he could speak and travel, but he had to maintain his grades.

And he did.

Ron's and my job was to outline the rules, and it was Justin's job to either abide by them or ask for help. Neither Ron nor I ever went online to check his grades. There was no need for us to check. Managing his grades was Justin's responsibility. If he failed a test, that was the natural consequence of his actions, and he would need to figure out how to fix it. Owning his problems was the key to his success.

Because Justin was leading assemblies at other schools, he often had to miss school to go speak. When we received a letter stating he had too many unexcused absences, we realized we needed a plan.

We called his principal and held a meeting with her. We were thrilled when she offered support. She had been involved with Justin's high school orientation and she knew his story. She also knew about all our fairs and the good, important work Justin was doing.

She agreed to let his speaking absences be excused as long as he made up all work, took his tests, and maintained his grades—in other words, all the rules we had already imposed.

Occasionally, we had difficulty with individual teachers. Thankfully, the principal, assistant principal, and guidance counselor had Justin's back, and they supported us every step of the way.

The Youth Ambassador program had provided Justin with a speech he used with success when speaking with teachers and younger audiences. With so many engagements, however, he knew he needed to do something a bit different—something that would reach middle and high school students.

The Youth Ambassador speech was also focused on Tourette Syndrome. As important as it was to educate about this condition, we knew there would not be a universal demand. Some schools would be interested in bully prevention, for example. This was a bit of a challenge, because we didn't like the word "bully." There was a time people could have called Justin a bully because of the way he acted. But that never entered our minds at that time. We also believed no one would stand up and say, "I'm a bully?"

The mission of our nonprofit focused on tolerance and self-acceptance. Some people criticized us stating that our beliefs were not enough. *They* wanted acceptance. Our position was that the concept of tolerance was a starting point. If we could get people to simply be tolerant of others and have respect, then everyone could begin moving toward the phase of acceptance. There were instances when we had to agree to disagree with people, and that worked. We held true to our values.

Justin set out to focus on this concept. He had many stories that demonstrated the intolerance he faced, and he could still educate about Tourette Syndrome by using his personal experiences. He wasn't quite ready to put his suicide attempts into his speeches, and Ron and I supported his decision.

Justin ultimately wrote a speech focused on being different. He told the story of the cross-country meet. He talked about the fairs and provided students with the idea that they could empower themselves by embracing their own differences.

"Embrace your differences" became his catch phrase.

———

CHAPTER 39

First Life Saved

Shortly after Justin started walking, he came to me and asked if I would officially become the Executive Director of his nonprofit. I was being hired by my fifteen-year-old son.

Although this was an easy decision, there were parts that were not as simple, including closing the company I built and grew for fifteen years. I didn't have the passion for it anymore. The feedback we were getting from people attending the fairs and speeches was the best drug out there—I craved more.

This meant I had to let people go. This was terribly hard, but unavoidable. It would also be a big financial hit. There was no way the nonprofit could pay me a salary anywhere near what I had been making. But this was not a financial decision; it was one of the heart. It was work I needed to do.

I officially became Justin's manager—the best decision I could make.

I began focusing on booking speeches.

One of our closest friends had a daughter at St. Francis Catholic School, and she offered to introduce me to the principal. When I called, she was interested and asked me about Justin's fee.

Fee?

I hesitated.

We never charged for his speaking.

We had never considered it.

I told her our goal was to have an impact on students and to share the message of tolerance and acceptance. She agreed to have Justin do an assembly for all her students in grades five through eight, and she explained firmly that they would donate to our nonprofit.

Justin began speaking at camps, leadership events, churches, and in local schools. Although we did not charge, most offered an honorarium.

Back when I started my promotional business, All Points Connect, it was done in an old-fashioned way. Before it was a business, I picked up the phone and made cold calls to see if I could drum up clients. It worked then, and it would work again.

I realized we needed to start charging a fee. Not only did we need the money, but the schools were receiving great value from the speeches. One of my biggest faults—still is to this day—is that I tend to undervalue myself. Now that Justin's and my livelihoods were intertwined, it was necessary to change all that.

Thanks to the Tolerance Fairs and media coverage, Justin's name was recognized in our community. Our next goal was recognition outside of our community.

In the fall of 2012, Justin was a sophomore. I started making random calls to schools outside of Cleveland to see if there was any interest. To my pleasant surprise, they took my calls, and more important, they were interested in the idea of a fifteen-year-old kid speaking to his peers.

Because my college roommate was in Cincinnati, I made calls there, and then I made a chance call to a private school in Baltimore. When I spoke to Erika at the Gilman School, we bonded. I told her we did not charge a fee but requested reimbursement for travel expenses. After a few conversations, we set a speech date for November.

Justin was going to do two speeches that day. One would be for the middle school and the other would be for their high school. This would be Justin's first high school audience and at a school outside of Cleveland. It felt strange that some of the kids would be older than him. It made me a little nervous but didn't faze Justin one bit.

The school paid expenses for both me and Justin, and we paid for Ron's travel. Erika graciously made our hotel arrangements and told us a car would be there to pick us up. We were happy to rent a car, but she insisted on taking care of us. I assumed we would call the driver when we arrived and would meet him at baggage claim.

Oh no—that was not how Gilman worked. As we walked toward baggage claim, we saw a dapper man dressed in a tuxedo holding a sign that said "Justin Bachman."

We looked at each other in total disbelief.

Was this us? Did that man really have our son's name on his sign?

Yes, he did!

Justin walked right up to him, extended his arm, and shook the driver's hand. We then proceeded to his large, spotless black Tahoe, and he told us stories of some famous people he had driven around.

We felt like royalty!

The speech Justin delivered was worthy of those fancy wheels, and he was immediately surrounded by students who wanted to meet him personally and take a selfie.

Shortly after we left the school, something unexpected happened. Private messages of thanks started rolling in, and kids were posting quotes and reactions on their social media pages. Some of the messages were rough. There were kids pouring out their hearts about difficult situations they faced. Many told Justin about the parts of the speech that struck a chord and would help them get through their difficult situations.

It just didn't seem real! But it was.

Justin continued to give speeches in the Cleveland area, and our next out-of-town trip came in March, when we headed to Cincinnati.

Anytime Justin spoke, Ron and I stayed in the back of the auditorium after the speech. This allowed Justin to interact with the students without us being on top of them. It gave the kids the ability to talk more freely.

At the engagement in Cincinnati, we noticed a beautiful girl hanging back from the crowd on stage. It was obvious she wanted to talk with

Justin but wanted to be the last one so she could have his full attention.

Sure enough, after the crowd dispersed, she approached Justin, and the two of them engaged in conversation for several minutes.

We will never forget what happened next.

I saw Justin put his arm around her shoulders and hug her. Then, they walked toward Ron. I was talking with a teacher. Justin introduced her to Ron and explained that she had a suicide plan. That morning, she came to school with her bookbag filled with some of her most prized possessions and she had been giving them away. Her intent was to end her life that night.

After hearing Justin speak, she had begun to question her decision, and she asked him if he ever had similar feelings. He told her he had, and he shared his journey. She started to cry because she finally felt seen. Justin told her that we, his parents, had helped him and that he wanted to introduce us to her. He assured her we would know how to help.

The ironic thing was we had no idea about what to do. We asked her if she had a trusted adult and she thought of her guidance counselor. We told her we would go with her—that made her feel better. She didn't know how to do this on her own, but having support made all the dif-ference. We don't know what happened after that, but we do know the guidance counselor was prepared and happy to help.

Then it happened again.

At Justin's next speech, another student approached him saying he had a suicide plan. Another child described cutting themselves to relieve the pain they felt. Thank goodness these kids were coming forward, but it was hard to learn about so much pain.

Ron and I realized we needed help in understanding how to handle these types of situations. With the demand for Justin's speaking rising considerably, we knew he would be approached by more students facing similar feelings of worthlessness and that included suicide.

We made two appointments. The first was with a nonprofit called Frontline. They were part of the national suicide prevention hotline and provided local counseling services. They gave us a wealth of information about resources available to kids who were having these feelings. We were thrilled to learn they had both a phone number and a texting feature for kids who were more comfortable reaching out via text.

We also met with a psychologist I had seen during Justin's darkest hours. She helped us create a protocol for the types of situations we were encountering at Justin's speaking engagements and gave us a line of questioning and the appropriate language to use. One of the most enlightening things she explained was the difference between the phrases "You need help" versus "You deserve help." It seemed subtle, but we soon realized there was a huge difference.

When you tell someone that they need help, they won't agree. They won't see the need. But the word "deserve" lets them know they have worth and are entitled to help. This was a big shift, and it reminded us about the ways in which we had to relearn how to speak with Justin. After leaving her office, we felt empowered and better prepared. I went on to be trained to sit on a suicide prevention hot line, which would come in handy over the next few years.

This was a real turning point for all of us. Justin realized the huge opportunity he had to make a difference. He decided it was time to write a new speech that included suicide.

CHAPTER 40

Living Loud, Can You Hear It?

Writing about his experience with suicide was emotional and difficult. There were memories Justin had blocked, and he needed to decide how far he wanted to go with the story. Ron and I did a lot of listening but knew anything Justin would say in his speech would have to come from his heart.

After many conversations, he decided to let people know he had made suicide attempts and to discuss the "why" but not the "how."

We were fortunate to meet two amazing speakers who offered to coach Justin. The first was David Coleman, better known as The Dating Doctor. David is a highly accomplished national speaker on the college circuit. He spent some time with Justin to help him create his new speech. Together, they added some interactive components, and David talked a lot with Justin about engaging the audience.

We also had a longtime friend, John DiJulius, an accomplished businessperson who built his business and reputation on customer service. John was a charitable and generous person. After hearing about Justin's speaking, he called and offered to help. John gathered his team together, and Justin did his speech for them. After hearing it, they brainstormed and offered suggestions on what moved them and where he might include more information. John also worked with Justin on making his entrance and holding the attention of the audience.

Justin went home, sequestered himself for a few days, and emerged with a new speech: Living Loud: Can You Hear It?

Justin debuted Living Loud on the road. One of our neighbors had moved to the New York City area, and her mom called to let us know they were planning her daughter's Bat Mitzvah and for her project, she wanted to raise money to have Justin speak at her school.

We were so honored and knew this would be the perfect place to present the new speech. We of course waived the fee, but they paid our travel expenses. We stayed in their beautiful home and had an incredible experience.

The speech was a huge hit! And the school took it one step further. We had worked with the administrators beforehand to prepare topics. And after the speech, they divided the students into small groups to discuss and further process the message. Each session was led by a teacher. Ron, Justin, and I split up so we could sit in on some of the conversations.

In one room, a teacher told a moving story about a boy who bullied her because of a skin condition when she was in high school. The boy told people she had leprosy and you could catch it by hanging out with her. She told the students how she dealt with the loneliness and isolation, and the story became a valuable lesson. The students saw their teacher as more of a human that day. It also gave them the courage to be vulnerable and share their own stories.

We came home from New York with a glowing recommendation from the school and a plan to share the new message far and wide.

However, things were not all good.

Some bristled at the topic of suicide and said it had no place in conversation, let alone in a speech to students. There were those who worried that Justin's discussion of suicide would cause kids to consider taking their lives.

These opinions bothered me, but I had to let them be just that— opinions of others. For the most part, I handled all of this with grace, but there were a few sad and unfortunate incidents.

There was a family we had been close with for years. We attended gatherings and socialized together quite a lot. But one day, everything came crashing down when we learned they opposed Justin's speaking. The exact words to us were, "You are creating a freak show out of your son."

Then came the ultimatum.

The mom told us the talk of suicide was something she could not condone and either Justin had to stop speaking, or our friendship would end.

We said goodbye to what we thought was a solid friendship.

We never looked back.

Their loss.

By his junior year, requests for Justin to speak were coming in almost daily. We were traveling at least two weeks out of every month during the school year. Things slowed down in the summer, but there were camps and leadership programs that kept us on the road.

We had some pretty insane trips filled with adventures. We got lost in Washington, DC, and ended up in the parking lot of the Pentagon. We have no clue how we got there, but we got a great laugh out of it.

One of our craziest trips took us to Denver, then to Cincinnati, Florida, Boston, Connecticut, and then home. In between speeches, we met with families who had a child with TS or a student in crisis, or with kids who wanted to do special projects. We made it a point to meet with anyone who wanted to meet with us, no matter the reason. We held true to our commitment of being there for anyone who may be feeling isolated or lonely. This enabled us to meet some incredible people!

The hardest part of all these trips was being away from Ron. Because he had his own company, if he didn't work, he didn't get paid. My salary was minimal, so we needed his. Occasionally, he would travel with us, but for the most part, the phone was our best friend.

On one of our multicity trips, Ron met us in Orlando. Justin was keynoting an educational association conference at the Dolphin Hotel on the Disney grounds. We had one free afternoon and decided to visit Epcot. We had from 2:00 pm until the park closed. We zoomed through and hit almost every ride. It was epic! We made the most of the little time we had. As it turned out, Boyz II Men was playing a live concert in a small nearby venue, so we got to see that too.

We made amazing memories.

Through all of these trips, Justin and I had created a well-oiled machine. I had my jobs for set up, and he had his. We had routines that included singing together in the car, and we sang and danced before every speech. At his speaking engagement, Justin required that his playlist be played as the students walked into the auditorium—to let the students know this was not your run-of-the-mill assembly. The two of us would stand in the back and dance to our heart's content. It got Justin psyched and ready, and bonding was so much fun!

I loved every second of it.

By this point, Justin really had "grown into his skin," and although the life he was leading was so different from what other kids were doing, he was going through the same types of emotions. He was beginning to like girls and have all the confusing feelings that hit boys in high school.

I felt so lucky that Justin would share his feelings with both Ron and me. We knew when he liked someone and helped him process the scary idea of asking girls out on dates.

Throughout high school, he had his share of crushes, but they never turned into anything. It was hard to watch him be hurt when the girls did not return his affections. He took one girl to a movie, and she picked *The Notebook*. That was their one and only date. We still give him flack for agreeing to see a "chick flick."

We treated these conversations as private and held them close to the vest. We could never risk breaking his trust. Justin needed to know we were the safest people to talk with about any problem he was facing. We did this with all our kids. When you prove you keep their confidences, they open up.

Justin was asked to keynote for some nonprofit and corporate organizations. He was invited as a panelist, and people were nominating him for more awards. One of the best awards he won was through an organization called the We Are Family Foundation. They ran a program called Three Dot Dash. Every year, they selected approximately thirty students—half from the US and half from other countries that they called Global Teen Leaders (GTL). They bring the GTLs to New York City for a week of leadership training and career-building experiences. On the last day of the program, they match the students with a mentor to help them grow their own organizations.

We are so thankful for Justin's experience with Three Dot Dash. He met some of the most incredible people and developed lifelong relationships. They truly became a family. Justin's mentor, Karen, was a gift. She provided the objective opinion we needed on how to grow the nonprofit. Karen challenged us to think in new ways. She was never afraid to tell us something we didn't want to hear. Thankfully, we were smart enough to listen!

Karen made connections for Justin and got him several prestigious speaking opportunities. One of the most meaningful was at a conference in Orlando called Sapphire. Software giant SAP held the conference every year, and over 25,000 of their customers attended. As part of the conference, the CEO, Bill McDermott, had an invitation-only day for about 300 executives. Karen and the team at Three Dot Dash asked Justin and one other Global Teen Leader to speak as part of Mr. McDermott's special day.

Justin was upstairs in his room when he received confirmation he would be speaking. He did his famous bolt down the stairs to share the news.

But this was different.

After giving me the details, Justin took a deep breath, looked at me, and said, "Mom, I want to go to this one by myself."

So many thoughts raced through my mind.

How could he not want me to go?

We always travel together.

I don't want to miss this moment.

And that's when I realized I had to let him go.

This was not about me.

It was not my moment.

All of this happened in a flash of seconds. Justin had no idea what was whirling through my mind.

I was so proud of all that Justin had achieved. The enormity of the independence he had gained and the confidence he built was a glowing beacon.

My baby bird was flying. He wasn't leaving the nest yet, but his wings were spread wide.

I remember so clearly dropping him off at the airport. We got his carry-on from the back of the car, I hugged him, and he walked away. I snapped a picture of him walking away from me into the airport.

I cried.

But they were tears of joy, accomplishment.

This was a turning point.

CHAPTER 41

The Suicide Crisis

Justin's speaking was incredibly rewarding and difficult all at the same time—but clearly, it was a highlight of our lives. The hard part came in seeing the trouble so many kids were facing. They lived with high anxiety, so many fears, and so much intolerance.

We knew.

We had been there.

There was one speech Justin gave on a Wednesday at a middle school. The following Friday night, he was upstairs in his room shortly before dinnertime. I'll never forget the sound of his feet flying down the steps and the pure panic in his voice.

A female student had just reached out to him in a private message on Instagram. She told him her parents were not home and she had slit her wrist. As the blood was gushing out, she remembered Justin's words and decided she didn't want to die.

Our training immediately kicked in, and Justin and I handled the situation together. Her Instagram handle didn't contain her name, so we had to ask her for it. Justin continued to message with her, and we called 911 to get an ambulance to her home. Next, as we continued to message with her, we called her school's principal on her cell, and thankfully, she answered. She was able to notify the parents.

Once the paramedics arrived, they took over and the messages stopped. Justin, Ron, and I stood together and held each other while we cried. We were calm during the storm, but once it subsided, the rush of emotion came rolling out.

We felt good that we had provided help.

We were so sad for this young woman.

What would have happened to her if she had not heard Justin's speech?

What if she had no one to call?

Would she have succeeded in taking her life?

Although difficult, this crisis was a reminder of the importance of our work and the difference we were making.

We had to keep going.

This doesn't happen often, but this young woman reached out a little over a year later to thank us and let us know she had gotten help and was doing well. More tears of joy flowed easily!

Questions.

Messages.

Personal stories.

Angst.

Came after all Justin's speeches.

Every single time.

My favorite part was the question-and-answer session he did at the end of every presentation. The audience questions were truly profound and reflected the anxiety students were experiencing.

One of the toughest questions Justin was ever asked was, "What's the most selfish thing you ever did?" Although I didn't agree with his answer, it came from his heart. Justin always knew where I was in the audience. I would give signals so he could find me quickly, no matter where I moved. He looked right at me as he answered: *what he had put us through as a family.* He told the students he didn't mean it, but that all his struggles felt so big, and he wished he had been more open to getting help sooner.

I knew Justin and I would have a long conversation about this later, and we did. I felt strongly about it, because I did not believe that what he did in the past was selfish. Many people believe suicidal people are selfish.

They are not.

To a person in deep despair, suicide feels like their escape. Their only relief. People with suicidal thoughts have distorted thinking and believe with all their heart that they are a burden. They assume that once they are gone, it will bring peace to their family. They don't consider the sadness their family will feel.

Suicide is not a selfish act.

Students asked Justin how to handle it when a friend expressed feelings of suicide. Our training told us to always inform the students that going to a trusted adult was the best help they could give their friends. Although it felt like a betrayal of friendship, it was the opposite. Kids are not equipped to handle helping a friend with deep depression and suicidal thoughts.

They asked about bullying and how they could feel good about themselves. Some students secretly confessed to being a bully and would ask about how to make things right. These children didn't feel good about themselves, and they needed to know how to turn that around.

All of this was hard on Justin. He internalized each question he received, and he wrote back to every single person who reached out. We knew we could not solve their problems and took the stance of letting the questioners know they were not alone and that we cared about them. We always told them they deserved happiness and that there are helpful resources available.

Some of the schools asked me to speak. Some wanted me to do a parent presentation, and others wanted Justin and I to speak together. Occasionally, a father's perspective was requested, and we were always thrilled to welcome Ron to the stage.

I enjoyed the opportunity to speak and experience the "high" Justin felt from the incredible reception from the audience. It is always rewarding to have someone approach us after a speech to let us know something we said resonated with them.

Applying to College

At the start of Justin's junior year in high school, college was on our minds. But Justin had other ideas. He wanted to take a gap year so he could speak full time. He was in great demand, and he wanted to take full advantage of the opportunity.

Ron and I had other plans. We held firm to the decision that Justin needed to go to college. I knew he would benefit more from going away and being on his own. Justin and I were spending so much time together, which was great, but it was not fostering his independence. He had to learn to fend for himself.

More important, he needed to experience his peers one on one and make friends. Although he managed his school schedule and held down a parttime job at the local ice cream parlor, I'd been managing his life schedule. It was time Justin learned about balancing life with school, finding your meals—all the responsibilities that would come with living on his own.

Although he was not thrilled with our decision, Justin acquiesced.

Justin thought that broadcast journalism might be something he'd like to pursue. He'd had a lot of exposure to various media outlets and had been interviewed by print, radio, and TV reporters. He struck up a wonderful relationship with the lead anchor for the 6:00 news on our NBC affiliate station—Russ Mitchell. Russ was so good to Justin. He had a special segment called "7 Minutes with Russ," where he engaged national and local leaders in a casual conversation. We were so humbled and honored when Russ asked Justin to be featured on a segment! It was a huge thrill, and it gave Justin the broadcast journalism bug—so when researching schools, he looked at colleges that had strong broadcast programs.

I'm not sure why, but Justin had his heart set on going to the University of Texas—*Hook 'em horns!* Ron and I didn't want Justin to put all his eggs in one basket, so we suggested he pick a few other schools so he could compare. He chose to look at Indiana University, Northwestern, and Michigan State. But we would head to Texas first.

There were no direct flights, and the connecting plane was a small puddle jumper, so the end result was a whole day of flying. *Strike 1.*

The Austin airport is cool and has some amazing art that gave it an energetic vibe. *Check!*

Because we arrived late in the day, we went to a restaurant recommended by a friend that claimed to be the best BBQ. It was! *Check!*

We went to sleep with great anticipation for the visit the next day. When we arrived on campus, we went to the admissions office and were broken up into smaller groups to go with student tour guides. Our guide was not exactly what you would call helpful. He told a lot of bad jokes and didn't give us the information we needed. He ended up asking everyone to donate money in way that made things uncomfortable. *Strike 2.*

As we walked around, we realized that although this was one of the biggest universities in the country, the actual footprint was small. The sidewalks were crowded, and there was little green space. We were constantly physically bumping into people. We could see Justin getting agitated, and his tics were increasing and his shoulders slumping. *Strike 3.*

University of Texas was out. It is a great school—just not for our son.

Justin was so bummed. He had been certain he would be a Longhorn—he had t-shirts and shorts, and this was supposed to be his new home for four years. It was an emotional moment. At this point, he still wanted to take off a year to speak, but his mean parents had said no.

Coupling this with the loss of a dream college experience, he was sad and angry simultaneously.

Ron and I had learned that the best thing to do was to leave him alone and let him process through it. This was still hard for me, because all I wanted to do was hold him and comfort my baby. But he wasn't a baby, and he had every right to be upset.

We essentially spent the evening in silence and then headed to our next stop, which was the Tourette Syndrome Association Conference in Washington, DC. This was our saving grace because Justin would be training a new group of Youth Ambassadors—one of his favorite activities. We would turn our attention back to the college search the following week. We were thankful we had advised Justin to review other schools.

We especially loved these conferences because we were able to be with friends who lived in cities across the country. I was having a conversation with our friend Autumn, telling her about our experience in Texas. She suggested we take a look at Syracuse, stating their Newhouse School of Public Communications was one of the best in the country.

Ron, Justin, and I talked about it and decided we would put it on the list. We couldn't add it to our upcoming trip because it was in a different direction, so we would do it the following week.

We visited Michigan State next, and from there, we went to Northwestern. Although they were both beautiful campuses with wonderful programs, Justin simply didn't have the "I can picture myself here" feeling.

We drove on to Bloomington, Indiana, and toured Indiana University. Because they did not have the exact major Justin wanted, we made an appointment with a counselor. Indiana was known for allowing students to create their own majors. Justin clicked with the person he met, and he was finally excited. He was going to apply, and this was his top choice.

Because he loved it so much, he didn't want to visit Syracuse and asked to cancel the trip. But the research we did showed great strength in the program, so we urged him to at least check it out. Although he agreed to go, it was with the understanding that no matter what, he was not going to like it.

When we arrived, his attitude was bad. We drove up late in the day and arrived for a late dinner. Because we didn't know our way around and it was dark, we ended up having a mediocre meal at a chain restaurant. This only confirmed Justin's decision not to attend this school.

He pouted and was crabby, but Ron and I knew to "ignore the noise." We continued to be upbeat, even though we wanted to lash out and give him an attitude adjustment!

The next morning, we went to the center where the tour would be held, and Justin was quiet and disinterested. Ron and I were pretty frustrated with his bad attitude, but we let it roll. We took a seat in the auditorium. The first speaker came out, and she was fantastic. Justin had been slumped in his chair and slowly but surely, he started sitting up. He was paying attention and hanging on her every word.

As we walked the campus, he livened up and bonded with the student guide who was in his major. At the end of the tour, Justin looked at Ron and I and said, "this is where I'm going to school."

It took everything I had not to say, "I told you so!" and inside, I had a giant smile he would never see!

We were all impressed with everything. There were beautiful green spaces, and many of the buildings had a Harry Potter feel on the outside but had the latest and greatest modern technology on the inside.

The toughest thing we learned was that the school of communications would be hard to get into. Justin wanted Newhouse and fortunately, we were able to secure a meeting with a counselor. This counselor made one thing clear: the program typically opened during the junior year; however, the school would take approximately 300–350 students as Freshmen direct admits. Although it wouldn't be a graduate-level degree, it would be the equivalent. The issue was that over 4,500 students would apply for these spots, so acceptance was competitive.

We were told that the best way to get in would be through early decision. This meant a firm commitment—if he was accepted, he was going. No brainer—the kid was hooked. We were also told that it would help to get a letter from a trustee in addition to the two letters of reference he needed from school and a professional relationship. We didn't know any trustees.

But that never stopped Justin before.

The first two letters were easy. He asked his government teacher—the amazing Rob Rivera—and Russ Mitchell to write letters. Russ had graduated from Syracuse's rival school, and at the end of his recommendation letter, he wrote, "I wanted Justin to go to my alma matter, but I guess you can't win them all." We got a good laugh out of that one!

Justin went on a quest, and he found ways to get to the people he needed. It's all about asking questions. We started asking everyone we knew if they knew someone who had gone to Syracuse.

You never know when the Universe will line things up.

Because Justin had recently won the Stop the Hate contest, he was asked to read his essay at the organization's major fundraiser. There were many influential people in attendance. While we were waiting for Ron to bring up the car, a man approached Justin to congratulate him. Because Justin asked him questions, he learned this man's architecture firm did work on some of the buildings at Syracuse University and he was friends with a trustee! This incredibly generous man—who did not know Justin but heard him speak—was willing to make an introduction.

Wow.

After another speech, a man approached Justin to tell him about an attorney he was friends with who lived in Syracuse and happened to be president of the Syracuse University Alumni Association. He too was willing to make an introduction. That would be two people!

And one of Ron's college buddies went to law school at Syracuse and was friends with a second trustee.

Networking worked!

Plans were made for another trip to Syracuse so Justin could meet with all three of these people. He would need to ask them all for the favor of a letter of recommendation. Each meeting was better than the next, and all were willing to do anything they could to help Justin gain admission.

Within a week, we had letters in hand, and Justin submitted an early decision application.

Then, we waited.

And waited.

There is nothing more stressful than waiting on a college decision when you want it so badly!

The date of acceptance notification was December 15. Justin was told he would get an email, which would be followed up by a written letter. We were nervous wrecks throughout the entire day.

We heard every second tick off the clock.

No message came.

Justin was devastated.

He went into his room to be alone. Because it was after 5:00, we were certain he had not been accepted. The sadness we felt was heavy.

Then, at 5:30 pm, the email came. The sound we heard was like a giant rumble of thunder as Justin bounced down the steps screaming "I got in!"

Justin was direct admitted to the Newhouse School of Public Communications as a Broadcast Journalism major.

We hugged and high-fived.

I was thrilled.

I was terrified.

How would we pay for this private school—we had no money. In fact, we were in debt up to our eyeballs.

This never stopped us before.

In the end, Justin would apply for forty-five scholarships. He earned enough to pay for most of his schooling, and he would become a resident advisor in his sophomore and years to avoid room and board costs.

Problem solved.

But the hardest question for me was—how was I going to let him go?

He was our last bird to leave the nest. When Stefanye left, we had the boys. When Konnor left, we had Justin.

But now?

Even though he had managed his Tourette Syndrome so well, would he be able to do it on his own without us there? What would happen if he had a problem with a teacher?

How would he live with a roommate he didn't know? This poor kid had no idea what he was in for!

In my heart, I knew he would be fine. He had grown so much and come so far.

He could do this.

He needed to do this.

I needed to let him.

I took great comfort in knowing we would only be a phone call away—or in the worst case, a five-hour drive.

Long ago, as we navigated the maze, we made a deal with Justin that he would always ask for help when needed it. He had honored his word, and I needed to remember that he would do the same while away at school.

We had done the basics. In our house, when the kids started high school, they started doing their own laundry. They all knew how to cook and manage money. Justin had been managing his medication for many years, so that was not an issue.

I faced the fact—Ron and I would be empty nesters.

That would be okay.

We would miss our children.

But it would be okay.

CHAPTER 43

Different Like You

The next year was a whirlwind as we prepared for Justin's college departure. We made the decision that I would run the nonprofit while Justin was away at school, and we would determine next steps when he graduated.

We made the very tough decision that he would not travel to speak while at school. He would still be able to speak during breaks, but this was going to be different.

We had received feedback that the name of our nonprofit was disconnected to the work we were doing. This led to the suggestion that we start doing business as "Different Like You."

I immediately loved this new name, but Justin was stunned—he didn't want it to change. Honor Good Deeds was his baby. It had been his salvation. It was his everything. He came up with the name, the mission, and he lived it. It was on his business cards and flowed so naturally every day.

This was hard for him. But the maturity Justin had gained as a person and as a businessman allowed him to process the change in exactly the right way. I could see the angel and the devil sitting on his shoulders.

This is the right thing to do.

This is not what I want.

Like everything, we talked about it. We went over every pro and every con. Justin continued to struggle.

We allowed him to struggle.

People tend to think struggling with something is bad. It's not bad, but it is hard. There is a huge difference. We learned that if we could embrace our struggles, it would give us the clarity we needed to work through it.

At first, Justin's response was anger—nope, no way. We let him be angry. His anger was his, not mine. In the past, I know I had gotten angry simply because he (or anyone else) was angry. But that is not a fair thing to do. It was my job to just listen and allow him to have his anger so he could work through it.

He ranted, I listened.

He asked questions, and they were calmly answered.

Then, he paused. He took his moment and walked away.

Justin came back and said he would go with the new name.

Although he had agreed, both Ron and I knew this was not easy for him. It was the right thing to do, and he had done it, but he didn't have to like it. His anger turned to sadness, which he also needed to process.

We had a number of conversations over the next few days and as each day went by, they became more nostalgic. We never took on Justin's emotions, but we were there, at his side to listen.

Within a few days, Justin was totally on board with our new decision and was ready to do the work to make the change effective.

One of our more exciting moments came with the development of our new logo. We were working with an agency, and their designer had come up with a number of concepts. When she revealed the "superhero," there was no need to go any further. Justin and I looked at each other and in unison said we loved it! It was awesome!

The figure was an orange outline of a person—gender neutral— hands on hips to show strength, and a flowing cape. This hero would stand strong in place of the letter "I" in the word "different."

We hired some consultants and began putting business processes in place. Our mission stated we were launching a website that was a safe, interactive, and life-changing outlet allowing users to discover immediate self-confidence and personal acceptance. Our goal was to educate to overcome ignorance, promote acceptance, and invite people to put Justin's message of "living loud" into action.

We had been holding fairs for the past three years, and we knew we had to mix things up in order to grow, so we decided to hold a conference. We would still engage our exhibitors and speakers, but we would also hold small, group breakout sessions. We learned we could engage teachers by providing continuing education credits they needed to keep up their licenses, and we went through all the necessary hoops with the schools to make it happen.

We created another student group to help us with the planning, led by our dear friend Erin, who was entering her junior year in high school. Justin trusted her fully and knew that when the time came, he could release the reigns to her.

Our Tolerance Fairs had always been free, but the conference was different. We opted to charge $25 to attend. This would include the full day of speakers, plus lunch.

The result was a fantastic lineup of presenters who spoke on topics ranging from dating advice and self-defense, to drug addiction and leadership training. We brought in both local and national speakers and focused on using students wherever possible. We had a panel of students that included a teen who had attempted suicide, another with an eating disorder, and one who was living in poverty to help inspire kids and let them hear from their peers.

It was easy to see that students who had attended our past fairs had come from some type of privilege—essentially, they had access to a car to get them where they needed to go and someone to drive them if they did not drive themselves. But we knew there was another group we needed to reach. And we knew this group would not be able to afford the conference fee, so we created a scholarship to enable them to attend.

Justin came up with the "60s Campaign." After running numbers, we realized it would cost us $60 for a student requiring transportation and lunch to attend the conference. Justin set to work to get funding and thankfully, this was an easy sell!

We received funding for 150 students, and we welcomed a total of 162 from Cleveland-area schools. We scheduled a number of busses to pick the students up at local recreation centers—places they could walk to and from. I'll never forget watching the buses unload on the day of the fair. The students were so excited to be attending—they were simply wonderful!

Seventy-nine teachers registered, and we could not be more thrilled. With other paying registrations, we had 350 people in attendance at our first conference.

One of the things we always preached to our children was the power of a handwritten thank-you note. We were so appreciative of our sponsors who enabled students to attend, we felt a handwritten thank-you was imperative. As the last item on the conference agenda, we provided paper and markers to all the students who had received a scholarship and asked them to write a thank-you note.

My original intention was to divide them up and send them to the sponsors. But after seeing the notes, I simply could not. I couldn't let go of them because they were so beautiful and so heartfelt. Many of them wrote that they knew they would never have been able to attend if it were not for their kindness. Instead of mailing the notes, I scanned them and emailed them to our sponsors.

The funny thing is that at no point, for all the events these organizations had sponsored, had they ever received notes, let alone handwritten ones! Each sponsor was so touched and grateful to receive them. They got to see firsthand the difference their donation made to this wonderful group of kids.

Once again, we basked in the glow of success. Watching hard work come together leaves the best feelings. Again, I closed my eyes to take it all in. I didn't know it at the time, but this would be our last event with Different Like You. I am so happy that I was intentional in remembering the special moments.

As we began the transition to me running the organization, we had to become more creative in developing programs I could manage that would still have a peer-to-peer component. Because we wouldn't have revenue from speaking, we had to identify other sources to drive funding.

We began developing leadership training and created a program that paired adult mentors with students. The work was rewarding, but could I sustain an organization founded by a teen designed to be peer to peer?

———

CHAPTER 44

Syracuse University

The day came, Justin was leaving for Syracuse.

We packed the car and hit the road. The Universe was again on our side. As we passed the first sign showing directions to the university, Justin's phone rang. It was the Administrative Assistant to Chancellor Syverud—the top guy! True to Justin's networking form, he had emailed the Chancellor a few days earlier in hopes of meeting him and now he was getting his chance. They scheduled something for the following week. They would end up having regular meetings, and Justin was one of two students (the other was a grad student) appointed to the Chancellor's committee for Diversity and Inclusion. They focused on making positive changes to the university culture.

Justin opted to participate in an early orientation program hosted by the university's Hillel organization. He got to move in ahead of the rush, and it provided a wonderful group of people to meet before classes started. They had students available to give personal tours of campus, and Justin felt like he knew his way around before school started.

When Ron and I had to say our goodbyes, I lost it. I thought I could hold it together, but I couldn't. All my worry came out in the form of big, ugly, gulping sobs. I held him so tightly that letting go seemed impossible. The weight of this moment was heavy—apparently it needed to be unloaded just like the U-Haul!

I was embarrassed, but it was so real that I just let it go. Of course, Ron and Justin thought it was funny and took pictures—wonderful… *not.*

Unlike me, Justin had no trouble saying goodbye. His excitement was evident, and he was ready to start this beautiful new chapter.

Seeing how quickly Justin got his bearings eased my mind.

Every kid should love college the way Justin loved Syracuse. He took advantage of all it had to offer. In addition to the Chancellor's committee, Justin joined a group called Orange Seeds. It provided leadership training and the opportunity to do community service every week throughout the year. It culminated in a big event. He made wonderful friends and expanded his social life.

Syracuse offered students the opportunity to live in Learning Communities—dorm floors centered around common themes and interests. Justin selected the leadership learning community, and he attended regular events and had students to study with.

One of my biggest worries was for Justin's roommate. After staying in many hotel rooms with Justin, I know he tics in his sleep, and it can be difficult to fall asleep when someone is making random noises. I'll call Justin's roommate situation "fine." They didn't become friends, but they were able to live with each other, which was a big relief. After his Freshman year, Justin would become a Resident Advisor during his sophomore and junior years, which gave him a private room in the dorms.

Justin joined a fraternity, which opened his world even more. It was nice to see him dealing with typical kid struggles again. Although he made some lifelong friends, there were those whom he didn't exactly jive with, and he had to figure out how to coexist in a living space with someone he didn't like.

Justin became an officer on the Interfraternity Council as the Director of New Member Education. Not missing a beat, he jumped back into nonprofit mode. He created a full curriculum that would be required for any new fraternity pledge. They would learn from experts about responsible drinking, race and privilege, the dangers of hazing, and sexual assault on college campuses.

Occasionally, my phone would ring when he needed to vent. He would rant—get it all out—then he'd say, "So how are you?"

I would laugh. I always loved the deep conversations we would have while traveling, and I was so relieved that we were still able to have them.

During his sophomore year, Justin met his first girlfriend. I drove up to Syracuse to get him, and I noticed he was wearing a turtleneck—Justin never wore turtlenecks. They set off his tics. Mom intuition told me he was hiding something. There were other friends around, so I didn't say anything, but the minute we got in the car I opted for humor. I sent him and Ron a text message that said, "Justin has a hockey." Thanks to spellcheck, my joke was even funnier!

We burst out laughing.

All my worry about Justin struggling was for naught. He was able to manage his course load, was busy with activities, and had a wonderful circle of friends. Although a bit of an overachiever, Justin was living a typical college student life.

We saw that the foundation we built for Justin was rock solid. That's when mine started crumbling.

CHAPTER 45

Time for Change

A few days after we returned home from dropping Justin off at school, I received a phone call from a woman who attended our first fair back in 2011. She had recently relocated to Atlanta and was working for SunTrust Bank. They wanted us to hold Tolerance Fairs for their employees in three cities—Atlanta, Georgia; Richmond, Virginia; and Baltimore, Maryland.

With Justin away at school, I was running Different Like You on my own. This news was fantastic and allowed us to continue our national focus. I got to work but quickly realized the request for this fair was different. The audience was all adults, and I didn't have our teens or Justin to rely on for help. I'm pretty nimble and an experienced event planner, so I used our model to plan three adult based Tolerance Fairs. I called Justin a lot, because that was what I always did when I needed a sounding board. Thankfully, SunTrust was thrilled with the events.

Right around the time SunTrust called, I received a request for Justin to speak at a conference for the Tourette Syndrome Association of Canada. Unfortunately, he couldn't attend because of school commitments, so I suggested that Ron and I speak instead. They said *yes!* I also told them I could find another student speaker and called one of the mothers we knew from Justin's days as a Youth Ambassador trainer, Nancy Brady, who said her son, Dylan, would be interested. Ron and I were thrilled to call Justin to tell him this amazing news. We relished the fact that Ron and I would be classified as international speakers before Justin had the chance!

We all got a great laugh out of that.

The conference was in Niagara Falls, which was an easy drive for us. When Justin won the Stop the Hate contest, as part of the decoration, they'd made life-size replicas of the ten finalists. We opted to bring cardboard Justin with us to the conference so he would be represented.

The speech we gave was wonderful, and many parents came up to us afterward to ask questions. Although it wasn't my first time speaking, it was the first time without Justin there. I desperately missed him.

I had a few more opportunities to speak, and I truly enjoyed them all. One of my favorites was for the Cleveland chapter of the Society for Human Resource Managers. There were more than a hundred people in the room, and I received a standing ovation.

Things were great, but there was an undercurrent of sadness I was having difficulty identifying.

Running the nonprofit on my own was different. I was working with a few schools on some customized programs, and we were doing a project with a Title One school that paired football players with mentors. Although these programs were rewarding, it was starting to feel like work—a feeling I hadn't experienced since we'd started the nonprofit. I was beginning to realize that running Different Like You without Justin was not for me. I could not find the energy to approach my days with the same determination I once felt. I was passionate about the mission, but I came to realize that this truly was Justin's organization. It's not that I wasn't doing a good job; I was. But it didn't carry the same joy that had come in the two of us doing it together.

But how could I tell Justin?

I remembered how difficult it was when we told him we were changing the name of the nonprofit. How would he feel if I said I thought we should shut it down?

How could I tell him I was not the person for this job?

I couldn't.

So, I pressed on.

When Justin came home for the summer, one day became particularly difficult for me. I can't remember what triggered my meltdown, but all of my feelings came barreling out.

Then, Justin said something that never dawned on me. He told me that while he was at school, my calls were always business related and he wanted his mom back.

We talked more, and I confessed that I was unhappy. Justin confessed that he was loving his broadcast classes and he needed to step away from the nonprofit. We agreed that we had done incredible work together, but we both needed to move on. It was time for Honor Good Deeds, doing business as Different Like You, to close.

We went out on top.

CHAPTER 46

Life in the Middle...

During Justin's early years, we lived life at the lowest point. Every day was dark and painful. Then, after years of navigating the maze, we'd lived a life of the highest of highs and everything was wonderful.

Neither is sustainable.

When anyone asks Ron how he is doing, he typically responds with, "living the dream."

He is right! The years felt like a dream. We were not without issues or sadness, but in the grand scheme of things, life was amazing.

We were saving lives!

At the start of 2017, Honor Good Deeds, doing business as Different Like You, officially closed. We had finished up the last of our projects and that was it.

Over.

For the first time in my adult life, I didn't have a job.

This was tough because our organization had allowed me to focus on my passion and do good work. *We saved lives.*

How could I find something like it?

Being an action-oriented person, I knew I needed to step up—but instead, I shut down.

All I heard from the people I spoke with was doom and gloom: *You will never make the money you want. People only hire young people, and you're too old. You can't find a job this time of year. Expect to be out of work for a year or longer in this economy...*

I needed to snap out of it, use my tools, and get my butt in gear!

How would I start?

In the past, my decisions were driven by others.

When I was growing up, my identity was as my parents' daughter. I was a shy kid, living in the shadow of a good-looking athletic brother and a cheerleader sister. My controlling parents chose my college and major.

Then I was Ron's wife. We married immediately following graduation, got jobs, and went to grad school, where I slowly learned to focus on things I enjoyed.

Then, I became Stefanye's mom, Konnor's mom, and Justin's mom. Don't get me wrong—I was (and still am) thrilled to be their mom. Even through all the difficulties, there was not one second when I did not love being a wife and mother.

My decisions were defined by my circumstances. I started my event-planning business, All Points Connect, so I could be home to take care of Justin. I took the position with the nonprofit so I could help Justin.

Again, I loved doing these things and have zero regrets, but they were never decisions made for me.

I needed to figure out how to live life in the middle.

No staggering lows.

No euphoric highs.

Just a nice, stable life right in the middle.

Good days, bad days, but no extremes.

It sounded kind of nice.

It was time for me to focus on me.

My birthday was approaching, and my tendency was to downplay it—but not that year. I was turning fifty-five, and I reflected on something Stefanye had done during college: she had the word "believe," along with Justin's initials, tattooed on her foot. It served as a reminder that you can overcome anything if you have faith. I loved the thoughtfulness she put into that, and I knew I wanted to do the same thing. I had never been a fan of tattoos, and this was something I never considered. Until I did.

I went to Ron and told him I wanted to get a tattoo, and the look of shock and joy on his face was priceless! I designed it myself: a heart that looks like a mother holding her child. I put a semi colon at the base of the heart and used another heart for the dot. The semicolon stands for a pause, and I changed the dot to a heart as a reminder to pause with love during difficult circumstances. I wanted the color to be teal for Tourette Syndrome. I placed this on my left wrist—the arm closest to my heart—where I would see it every day.

Something about that tattoo helped me move forward. It reminded me of my own significance and success as a caregiver. I know I'll never forget my past, but this was a constant reminder of my biggest life accomplishment. With all the kids out of the house now, I could focus on me. I could make my own career decisions. But I needed to make them fast, because we needed an income.

Our finances were tight. We had taken out a second mortgage to pay Justin's medical bills, so we had a mountain of debt. Ron was working, but as a one-person business, his income potential was limited. We had made choices long ago to focus on our family. They were the right ones but left us with financial issues. Ron always liked to call us the wealthiest family that had no money.

The biggest problem was that I had no idea what to do. I had worked for myself and at home for many years. I had done so many different things that figuring out exactly what my next step would be was challenging.

I turned to my kids, who were excited to help me, and we had some enlightening conversations.

"I have no idea where to start or what I want to do."

Stefanye told me, "Mom, yes you do! Take your own advice and focus on the things you like to do."

Konnor said something similar. "Mom, you do you! Think about your strengths. You need to reintroduce yourself and focus on what you are good at doing."

And so did Justin: "Mom, yes you do! You are a branding expert. Go back to the branding exercise we did with Different Like you and do it for yourself!"

Funny how they all had the same great advice.

I took a personal inventory.

I am a problem solver. We were dealt a tough hand, but instead of looking at everything as insurmountable, my view saw challenges to overcome. I became resilient. When a problem arises, I acknowledge it, analyze it, and look for solutions. I am highly resourceful. Present me with a challenge, and I will attack until it is solved.

I'm also highly energetic and enthusiastic—always with a can-do attitude. I don't give up easily, and I love engaging in conversations that allow me to learn what makes people who they are. Everyone deserves to be happy, and if I can make that happen, I will.

My favorite brand component is my drive and passion to help others—personally and professionally. I learned early in my career that the client is king. I pride myself on getting to know my clients and learning how I can make them shine.

This exercise helped me remember who I was on the inside, and I felt ready to write a new resume.

It sucked. It showed what I did, but not what I accomplished.

Rewrite!

I was having many conversations with myself. Although I wanted immediate action, I knew things didn't happen overnight. The first draft is never perfect. I had to give myself permission to slow down. Most important, I had to remind myself that in the past, I'd gone through adversity but always landed on my feel.

No matter what, each storm ended, and the sun returned.

I went back to the drawing board.

Again, it was my kids and my husband who reminded me of my

accomplishments. They said things like, "Remember when *ESPN Magazine* ranked your team second in game entertainment in all of sports?" and "You built and managed a million-dollar company from the ground up and maintained the same staff" and "You have raised millions for a multitude of nonprofits."

I started to look at my job search as a project with goals and objectives. I needed strategy and tactics. The first thing I did was make a list. The list had names of people who were high-level influencers. As my husband likes to say, "it isn't always who you know, but who *they* know." High-level executives know people! I knew some of the people on my list, but there were more that I had never met. I did some sleuthing to find phone numbers and emails, and I worked the list. It was awesome! Almost everyone I contacted agreed to meet with me.

That same week, I received an invitation to a lecture at a local college. The speaker, Mr. Jeff Hoffman, was amazing. I listened intently. He posed the question, "What is your dream job?" He suggested writing each dream on a sticky note. He further instructed the audience place those notes in a highly visible spot where we would see them every single day.

I went home that day and wrote five notes, which I placed at the bottom of my computer screen. They said:

Be a speaker.

Work with pro athletes.

Support good causes.

Travel outside the US, especially to Australia/New Zealand.

Make $$.

I admit I was skeptical. Just because I wrote these things down didn't mean they were going to come true. I mean, seriously, that wasn't enough to make them happen, but I was willing to give it a try. These were lofty goals, but they were my dreams.

What I later realized is that when you make a goal that you see every day, you subconsciously start to look for things related to it.

I started the process of meeting people from my list. I went into each meeting knowing I needed something, but I was terrified to look desperate.

My first meeting was a disaster.

It was with a high-level executive at an ad agency. I had met her once before a few years back, but I did not really "know" her. She asked me what I wanted to do, and my answer was essentially, "I am good at a lot of things." She then asked me how she could help, and my answer was, "I was hoping you had suggestions for me."

My inner voice was loud and clear: "I'm blowing this." But I refused to panic and instead asked her how she would approach a job search. Best question ever, because boy, did I get great advice!

She told me I needed to do more homework. While she agreed I had held a lot of different jobs and had a vast array of skills, choosing something pertinent to the person with whom I was meeting was essential, and I needed a specific ask. For example, she was in the advertising industry. Had I done my homework, I would have researched the client list on their website and asked to be introduced to any of the nonprofit organizations they served.

I left her office a bit embarrassed, but just like those appointments with neurologists and psychiatrists, teachers and coaches, I learned something. I realized these meetings were not interviews but fact-finding missions. Maybe they would lead to a job, but more likely, they could lead to a recommendation. I relied on advice from my coach, Libby. She is a spiritual person and helped me understand that if something isn't meant to be, then something better is coming. This philosophy allowed me to use the meetings to get to know people and learn about their goals and objectives. After all, it was my responsibility as a job seeker to demonstrate how I could help their company.

Another friend suggested that I set up Google alerts. He told me these would help me see what's happening, know when jobs opened up, and learn valuable industry information. This was so helpful and led to me feel more in the know.

As the days went on, I realized I was having a blast. I was meeting some amazing people. If only I could make a living looking for a job!

The result? Within about two weeks, I landed a position with a company that did sports marketing for professional athletes. They hired me to help the athletes create events that would feed social media stories.

Chalk one up for my sticky notes: I was working with professional athletes!

The company was about to announce a partnership in Australia, and I would be involved. That hit sticky note number two!

The hiring manager told me they were in the process of securing funding and didn't yet have the ability to pay me. He asked if I would start as a volunteer and move to a full-time, paid employee within two months. The salary they were offering was well within the range of what I wanted.

I took the job.

Big mistake.

Never ever take a job without getting paid. I should have told them I would wait until their funding was secure. I ended up giving this job my all way past the date when they told me the position would be funded. I finally had a conversation with the CEO, and he was shocked when I said I would no longer work for free.

I had to chalk that one up to a major lesson. There was a part of me that knew in my gut I was not making the right decision—I should have listened.

I looked back at those notes on my computer and wondered what the heck I was doing. I had a mini breakdown. My pride was hurt; I felt damaged. All I could think about were the naysayers who told me what I could not do.

I had made a colossal error in judgement.

Could I trust myself?

I allowed myself a few days to boo-hoo, then remembered that this was nothing compared to the adversity we faced before. I paid special attention to another note I had put on my computer that said: "Don't give up, don't ever give up."

It's funny how we can be our own worst enemies and not see real opportunities that are in front of us. When you allow yourself to open your mind and really see, you will be amazed at what's out there.

I went back to the drawing board. Again.

I started a new job search.

Amid this, Ron and I got another of those calls no parent ever wants to receive.

Stefanye had been in a terrible skiing accident. The ski patrol had to put her on a sled to take her two miles to the waiting ambulance. She required emergency surgery that resulted in a metal plate and six screws. She had a complete break of the largest bone in her body.

Her fiancé, Matt, never left her side and kept us informed, which meant the world to us. Although we offered to fly out to Vail, he told us he had it covered, and would rather we help when they got home to Nashville.

The universe again lined things up. I was not working and had the flexibility to be there for our kids. Two days later, I flew to Nashville. Ron had to stay home and work, because we could not give up his income.

I would spend the next two weeks helping Stefanye and Matt. It was absolutely gut wrenching to see my daughter in so much pain. But it was also beautiful to see the love between these two kids. I missed Ron terribly, but we knew we were doing what needed to be done. And Stef and Matt were so appreciative.

Toward the end of my nursing duties, I received a call from one of the athletes I met at the awful job. He wanted to work with me directly. Stefanye had healed to the point where she could get around on her own, so I headed home to investigate this new opportunity. I'd been out of work for almost six months with no income. Even a little project bringing in some money would be helpful.

For a while, I continued to do project work, but nothing was touching my passion, and I was not earning enough to put a dent in our mountain of debt.

Our finances were getting worse, and we were near the point of being unable to pay our bills.

The only thing we could do was sell our home. This was sad. We loved our home. We designed and built it to have everything we needed. We had a beautiful, wooded lot that gave us privacy and it was big and roomy.

I could not yet pull this trigger. I felt so guilty and didn't want to do this to Ron. He loved the house, working in the yard—I just couldn't do it.

We had curtailed our social life—we didn't have the money to go out for dinner. Our lifestyle was changing completely because we didn't have the financial means.

To make matters worse, Ron was struggling physically. His body was telling him he had swung the hammer one too many times. His knees were giving him problems—too many trips up and down the ladder.

He was thinking about his next steps and wondering if he should close his business. But he couldn't do anything until I had a job because he was our only source of income.

We made the agonizing decision to sell our beautiful home.

We put our house on the market and began to discuss what we would do next. Our hope was that we could sell our home and pay cash for something smaller or move to an apartment. Our house had great value and many incredible features, but it was a difficult buyer's market.

I was mortified over our financial position and the fact that I was still doing project work and could not get my career on track.

One night, Ron was sitting upstairs in our loft, working on his computer. I sat down and, on a whim, asked him, "Why are we staying in Cleveland?"

He looked at me and replied, "I don't know."

We talked for a while, batting around the idea of why we were staying.

We had become complacent. We were hanging out with the same

people in the same places, doing the same things we'd done for years. We rarely exercised or did anything spontaneous.

All three of our kids lived in different states. Two of them were a plane ride away and one was a five-hour drive. None of them showed any interest in coming back to Cleveland.

We talked about our history, friends, and the network we had in Cleveland, but we also had friends and a huge network we had built across the country. In fact, the people I considered to be like sisters didn't even live in Cleveland.

We could stay in touch with everyone.

A big decision was made.

We were moving!

But where?

We had fun figuring this out. There were a few factors that would determine where we would go. We decided we were done with snow. We were still young, and we wanted to be outdoors more often. Next, we needed to be in a city that had a large airport so we could easily travel to see the kids. Finally, I always felt a pull to the ocean. I didn't want to live on the beach but did want to be someplace where we could easily get there.

There were lots of options—Florida, California, the Carolinas, Texas—many places to research.

Ron and I decided we would both start looking for a job and whoever landed one first would pick the city where we would move.

Because he still had to work, it was much easier for me to focus on the job search.

It's funny how things in your past plant seeds for the future. Through the failures I experienced over the past year, I learned a lot and was putting those lessons to work. I always knew the power of networking, but this job search took everything to an entirely new level. I began calling everyone!

Our son-in-law Matt had a friend who was working in the athletic department at the University of Central Florida. Matt made an introduction and I spoke with him. He had a friend who was a realtor and he introduced me to her. This realtor knew a person who worked for the Central Florida Foundation. I called this person, and she introduced me to a woman who was with the Edyth Bush institute. This woman suggested I call a local businessman who was on the Board of Directors for the Holocaust Memorial Resource & Education Center of Florida, where there was an open position.

He made an introduction for me to the Executive Director, and we scheduled a call. It was fantastic. She told me all about the organization and that she was looking for a Development Director.

While I was talking with her and she was outlining their plan, I immediately knew I wanted to pursue this. The only problem was that the next day, she was leaving on a three-week trip to Poland.

I was crushed—how could I wait that long!

The woman was upfront with me and said that while I sounded qualified, she needed someone who knew the Orlando market—who had connections. While I got that, I knew I could quickly make any connections I needed.

I knew that if I wanted this, I was going to have to make things happen. I needed to take initiative and go to Orlando. I lined up four interviews!

Then, I called the Executive Director from the Holocaust Center and told her I would be in town, would she be willing to meet with me? I told her I completely understood her concerns, but I asked for a conversation, and she agreed.

Sometimes, it feels like life throws things at you to make you shake your head. Right as I was planning my trip, I slipped and fell while mopping the floor. I ended up with a broken elbow and wrist. Really?

I was a bit nervous to travel on my own with two broken bones, but I put on my big-girl pants, and I did it. People were nice and helped me lift the suitcase into the overhead compartment.

It was the beginning of July. I would be traveling home on the July

Fourth holiday, which meant I would miss the fireworks celebration, but so be it. I was determined to come back with a job!

All my meetings were fantastic. I was so happy I'd made the trip. It was worth every penny we spent.

When I left the meeting at the Holocaust Center, the ED still had reservations about bringing in someone from out of state with limited connections. She told me she would really put some thought to it though.

While I didn't come home with an offer in hand, I had a feeling it was getting close.

The planets lined up—on August 15, we sold our house, and I received an offer.

It was meant to be.

We were moving to Orlando, Florida.

We decided to jump full in and do a complete downsize. We were committed to a new beginning—a total adventure!

We hired a company to do an online auction—our plan was to sell the majority of our belongings.

Packing up eighteen years of crap from three kids was daunting, to say the least. We were amazed at the things we found. Turns out I had a brand-new sewing machine that was never removed from the box! There was a fondue pot—never used.

All the kids came home, and together we strolled down memory lane. We found all the notes they had written to the tooth fairy, various apology letters, and a united movement to request a trip to Disney—oh, the irony in that one!

Before the kids left, we took a photo with all of us in front of the house. We drove around town to the Cleveland sign and took pictures with the downtown area in the background. It was an awesome way to say goodbye to a city we loved.

We worked for days from early morning until late at night to prepare items for the auction, pack, and clean. On the day of auction pick up, one by one, we saw our belongings carried out of the house.

We were left with our sectional couch, one TV, computers, photographs, some kitchen items, and a whole lot of memories.

We packed up my car and Ron's truck, and we hired a moving company for the couch and TV.

We took one last walk through the empty house and said a tearful goodbye to our next-door neighbors, whom we adored.

It was strange.

But it was good.

We got in our cars in the early afternoon of September 12, and we pulled into our new apartment in Orlando on September 13.

As I parked, out of nowhere, I burst into tears! The sun was shining and there were palm trees all around. I could not believe this dream had come true.

CHAPTER 47

Today

There is so much to like about Orlando! The weather is perfect, the nature is beautiful, and there is so much see. The restaurant scene is vibrant, and we have tasted food from many different countries. There is a thriving art community, and the diversity has broadened our world.

We are still living in our apartment, which is perfect for us. We committed to the most minimal way of life, and it's been great. It has given us flexibility to do more. We don't have yard work, and cleaning is quick and easy.

We frequent the beach all year round. We are regulars at our favorite restaurant, where I always enjoy oysters and a rum runner!

I'm so happy to be on this incredible adventure with my best friend in the whole world. And boy have we adventured! Every weekend, we have made it a point to do something fun. We step away from work, we go out, and we enjoy. During the pandemic, we pivoted to home activities like puzzles, walks, and movies.

We have made new friends.

Our family is thriving.

We are grandparents! Talk about pure joy. Stefanye and Matt are incredible parents, and we are so proud to watch them grow.

Konnor has a wonderful job and has quickly advanced in his career—he works in sports—which was always his dream.

Justin is now a broadcast journalist reporting the news. The kid with the tics is live on television! Thanks to the internet, we get to watch his stories.

There have been a few bumps—shit we never saw coming, like a pandemic and cancer, set us back—and we experienced those moments of self-doubt that always come when the chips are down. But we won!

Everything we have been through reminds me that the storms will always roll in. On some days, the thunder may be louder, or as big as a tornado or even a tsunami.

But no matter how big the storm, it passes.

The sun always returns.

It may take days…weeks…years.

But stick with it, work hard, ask questions, turn around, and find a new path. Life will get better.

Every day, Ron and I look back to remember how far we have traveled. It took me a while, but I learned we deserve every ounce of happiness life has to offer.

We are thankful for our family and for the journey.

All of us continue to give back. We know how much was given to us, and we have the joy of being able to pay it forward.

Every day, people are contemplating suicide.

At first, I was going to write that we were lucky.

But we weren't lucky.

Luck had nothing to do with it.

Hope had nothing to do with it.

Unconditional love kept us going.

It was persistence, and the drive to never give up that got us to where we are today.

We pulled together as a family—all of us. We worked hard, and that showed us the way out.

I know that so many people are struggling.

I never ever want anyone to go through or feel the loneliness our family felt during our darkest days. I hope you know you matter. Each and every one of us has the power to choose how we focus our energy, how we act and respond to what life sends our way.

I know firsthand that it is easy to feel helpless.

It sounds clichéd when people say, "You are not alone." In some ways you are—you are alone in your own experience. Only you can feel what you feel.

But I'm here to tell you, there are people around who can show up for you, who can help, but you have to let them.

I have made helping my personal passion. I still receive calls from families across the country who have a suicidal daughter, or are dealing with a son who feels different or has been diagnosed with a frightening medical condition, as well as many parents of children with Tourette Syndrome.

I promise to listen.

I hope the Bachman Gang's story resonated with you and makes your journey a tiny bit easier. If nothing else, please know you are not alone.

I'm right there with you.

A Father's Perspective

September of 2020 marked ten years since Justin's Bar Mitzvah—a milestone occasion in the life of any Jewish youth. The day you supposedly become an adult. As I have watched my son grow, I continue to be awestruck. A decade ago, we weren't sure that he would survive his demons and we didn't know if we would survive as a family.

Here are some observations from our journey through the maze:

- First and foremost, I am so thankful that we made it to the other side. My heart goes out to families that have lost a loved one to suicide. We came close but can never fully imagine that horrible pain.

- In the darkest of hours, find hope. Focus on the positive. While it doesn't always seem like there is any, find something. Even the smallest sliver of light can help you maintain some semblance of sanity. Do what you need to do to keep moving forward. If you don't take care of yourself (both physically and mentally), you can't begin to help someone else.

- Try to remember who is doing the work. While Lisa, Stefanye, Konnor, and I were there, it was Justin who bore the brunt of the effort. Lots of therapy for all of us, but the yeoman's lift was his. We were the supporting staff to his leading role. I'm not saying that it wasn't difficult for the rest of us (it was), but watching Justin muscle his way through the maze made me realize a lot about the whole big picture.

- Asking for help is not a bad thing; it's a good thing. We met a lot of people on our journey who tried to hide or were in denial about the mental health issues that they or a family member were dealing with. The negative stigma regarding mental health blew our minds. From insurance not covering procedures, to school programs not addressing it, to people just shying away from you when your family is dealing with a mental health issue—it is one of the biggest untold concerns we face.

- Mental health problems are ongoing. Therapy, correct medications and support systems all play a part in dealing with them, but they never go away. There may be a stretch where things are "good," but there may also be times when they aren't. Again, it's always okay to ask for help.

- I was amazed by how many people commented on how involved I was as a father. When we became involved in the Tourette Syndrome Association and started going to national conventions, I was usually one of a small handful of fathers in attendance. I don't know if it has to do with machismo, denial, or something else, but this always puzzled me. Dads, get involved!

- Listen to your child. They may be young, but they know of what they speak. It is easy to be dismissive—trust them when they tell you what they need.

- Everyone thinks they know what you are going through and will often volunteer their "expertise" on how to "fix" the problem. Try to ignore them, as this is just noise.

- You will probably lose people you thought were friends. The corollary is that you will find others you didn't know were your friends.

- Remember that we are all different. Our differences are what make us awesome. Learning to "embrace our differences" can change the way we look at ourselves, as well as the world in general.

- Finally, trust your gut. If you think a friend or family member seems "off," say something. If you haven't heard from someone in a while, check on them. Again, your gut feeling is right more often than not. It's better to check on someone and be told no than to not check on someone and….

- It's a scary crazy time in our world right now. Work to be part of the change that you want to see. As a wise person once told me: To the world you may be just one person, but to one person you may be the world.

I think I'm the lucky one. More tears of joy. Love you
Justin Bachman

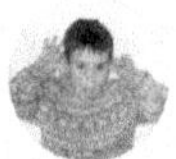

Justin Bachman is with **Lisa Bachman.**
May 12, 2019 ·

The only time you should ever look back is to see
how far you've come.

When I was 10 years old I looked my mother in the
eyes and told her I would not live to see age 18. I
had attempted suicide three times already and in
my mind that was a promise. She had other plans.

It's appropriate that I graduate on Mother's Day.
You are my inspiration, my rock, my shoulder to
cry on and my best audience and my wisest
advisor. You are why I'm here. Thank you for all of
our road trips, all the giggle, all fits the random
conversations in the kitchen that teach me about
life. We've shared tears both happy and sad, and
through it all I wouldn't change a thing.

Happy Mothers Day. For all the hell I put you
though, you never once backed down. You're the
best there is, and I don't know how the hell I got
so lucky. BGOD.

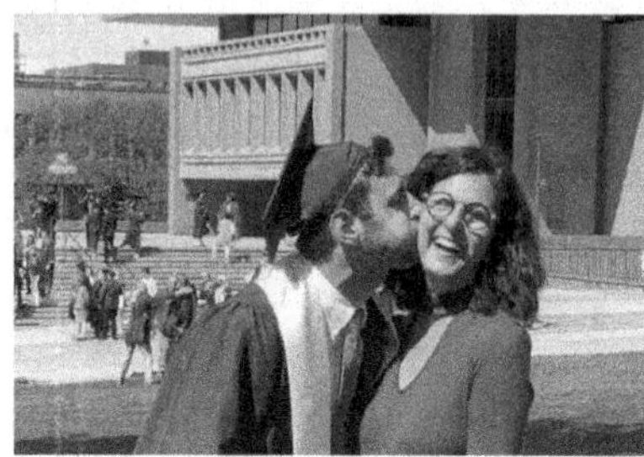

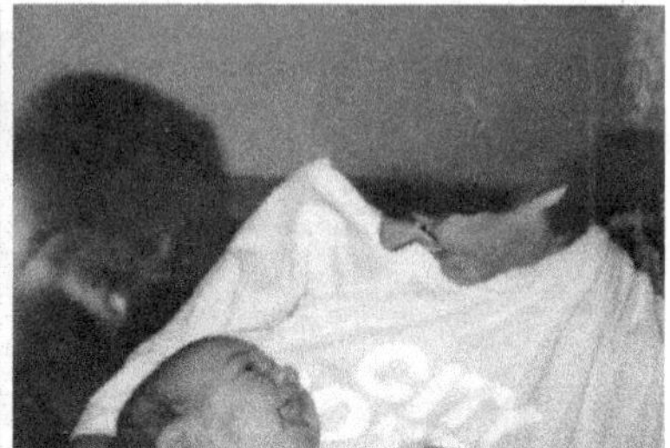

About the Author

Lisa Bachman is a proud and loving wife of thirty-six years, the mother of three grown children, and grandmother to two little boys (so far). Never a person to back down from a challenge, she takes on her most difficult tests with tenacity.

At the start of her career, she was a computer programmer, but realized she'd rather talk with people than machines, and rose through the corporate ranks becoming project manager at Progressive and then a top sales producer at Cisco Systems. When her youngest child was born, she found the corporate world unable to meet her needs, so she left and launched a non-traditional marketing agency called All Points Connect. For eighteen years, she grew this thriving nationwide organization. Lisa enjoyed a decade of relationships with brands such as the Cleveland Cavaliers, NASCAR, Dunlop Tires, Sherwin Williams, Clear Channel, General Mills, Liquid Nails, CBS Sports, AEG, and many others all while raising three children and dealing with her youngest son's mental health challenges.

When the call of her son's nonprofit—Different Like You—tugged at her heartstrings, Lisa closed her company to concentrate on those efforts full time for five years. Today, Lisa is the Director of Development and Marketing for the Giving Back Fund.

She is a published author and seasoned public speaker, focusing on topics ranging from raising children with differences, suicide prevention, Tourette Syndrome, volunteerism, non-profit organizations, and marketing. Lisa will always stop to talk with a person in need. She practices what she preaches both personally and professionally—striving to be someone who makes a difference and gives back as much and as often as possible. Lisa never wants anyone to feel as alone as she once felt.